Healing
Injuries
the
Natural Way

How to mend bones,
muscles, tendons
and more

Michelle Schoffro Cook

First published in Canada in 2004 by
Your Health Press ™, a division of Sarahealth Inc.
In association with Trafford Publishing.

IMPORTANT NOTICE:

The purpose of this book is to educate. It is sold with the understanding that the author and publisher shall have neither liability nor responsibility for any injury caused or alleged to be caused directly or indirectly by the information contained in this book. While every effort has been made to ensure its accuracy, the book's contents should not be construed as medical advice. Each person's health needs are unique. To obtain recommendations appropriate to your particular situation, please consult a qualified healthcare provider. The herbal remedies recommended in this book are for education purposes only and should not be used without consulting a qualified expert in herbal medicine.

Printed in Victoria, Canada

A cataloguing record for this book that includes the U.S. Library of Congress Classification number, the Library of Congress Call number and the Dewey Decimal cataloguing code is available from the National Library of Canada. The complete cataloguing record can be obtained from the National Library's online database at: www.nlc-bnc.ca/amicus/index-e.html
ISBN: 1-4120-3005-6

TRAFFORD

This book was published *on-demand* in cooperation with Trafford Publishing. On-demand publishing is a unique process and service of making a book available for retail sale to the public taking advantage of on-demand manufacturing and Internet marketing. **On-demand publishing** includes promotions, retail sales, manufacturing, order fulfilment, accounting and collecting royalties on behalf of the author.

Suite 6E, 2333 Government St., Victoria, B.C. V8T 4P4, CANADA
Phone   250-383-6864   Toll-free   1-888-232-4444 (Canada & US)
Fax   250-383-6804   E-mail   sales@trafford.com
Web site   www.trafford.com   TRAFFORD PUBLISHING IS A DIVISION OF TRAFFORD HOLDINGS LTD.
Trafford Catalogue #04-0832   www.trafford.com/robots/04-0832.html

10   9   8   7   6   5

OTHER BOOKS BY YOUR HEALTH PRESS ™

Stopping Cancer at the Source by M. Sara Rosenthal, Ph.D. (2001)
Women and Unwanted Hair by M. Sara Rosenthal, Ph.D. (2001)
Living Well with Celiac Disease: Abundance Beyond Wheat and Gluten by Claudine Crangle (2002)
The Thyroid Cancer Book by M. Sara Rosenthal, Ph.D. (2002)
Living Well with an Ostomy by Elizabeth Rayson (2003)
Thryoid Eye Disease: Understanding Graves' Ophthalmopathy by Elaine A. Moore (2003)

Soon to be released...

Pediatric Glaucoma and Cataract Disease: Your Questions Answered by The Pediatric Glaucoma and Cataract Disease Foundation and edited by Alex Levin, M.D., F.R.C.P., Director, Ophthalmology, The Hospital for Sick Children (2004)
Menopause Before 40: Coping with Premature Ovarian Failure by Karin Banerd (2004)
Coping with Molar Pregnancy and Choriocarcinoma by Tara Johnson and Meredith Schwartz (2004)

DEDICATION

I dedicate *Healing Injuries the Natural Way* to Curtis, my beautiful husband and soulmate. You're the best thing that ever happened to me and you've always been and will always and forever be my one true love.

CONTENTS

ACKNOWLEDGEMENTS

There are many people I'd like to thank for their support with my healing and help in making this book a reality.

First, I am eternally grateful to my husband Curtis. You're the reason this book happened at all and also the reason that I have healed so much. Thank you for your unconditional love, even in the face of massive obstacles. Thank you for all the ways you supported me while I wrote this book—for the massages, Reiki and biofeedback treatments you gave me as well as the healthy foods and juices you prepared to help me overcome my injuries. You're an inspiration.

Thank you to my parents, Michael and Deborah Schoffro, who've always motivated me to continue with my writing. Your support, love and friendship mean a lot to me.

Thank you to Harvey Diamond, for providing the Foreword to this book and for pioneering the movement to use food as medicine. I credit Diamond with inspiring countless people (including me) to search for a natural solution to health concerns.

My gratitude also goes to Dr. Carri A. Drzyzga. You were a tremendous support on my healing journey, a wonderful person whose friendship I value, and a fabulous expert reviewer for this book.

As well, I thank Dr. Robert Laquerre for taking the time to get to the bottom of my pain and suffering. Your patience and support made a huge difference to the quality of my life.

Thanks to my sister, Bobbi-Jo Meyer, and brother-in-law, Rick Meyer, for constantly pestering (I mean, motivating) me to eat a largely raw diet.

Thank you to Sara Rosenthal, Larissa Kostoff, and Laura Tulchinsky, the team at Your Health Press ™. You've been a pleasure to work with.

And many thanks to everyone else who helped or supported me. You know who you are.

PUBLISHER'S PREFACE

*H*ealing *Injuries the Natural Way* resulted from many emails from browsers to *www.sarahealth.com* (and readers of my own books) requesting that Your Health Press ™ "do a book" from the perspective of the alternative health movement about complementary healing for fractures, muscular problems, soft tissue injuries, and so on. We learned that many people suffering from an array of injuries lived their lives feeling unwell, often years after a specific injury had been treated. We also recognized a growing need to cover the topic of injuries as our population ages.

As of this writing, we are facing in North America a virtual epidemic of dependence and addictions to prescription pain medications in particular. The majority of these addictions begin because people are seeking remedies for pain caused by common debilitating conditions associated with aging, or specific injuries. Many injuries occur as a result of normal, repetitive tasks that take their toll as a result of bone loss, arthritis, and aging bodies. Living with pain can reduce mobility and independence to such an extent that legitimate pain management can lead to the slippery slope of addiction, where the body becomes increasingly more tolerant of chemical pain relief, creating the need for higher or more frequent doses.

According to the National Institute on Drug Abuse, from 1990 to 1998 the number of new users of pain relievers increased by 181 percent. Since the last statistics were recorded, these numbers have significantly increased. For the first time, a recent request for research by the National Institutes of Health (NIH) has gone out to medical and behavioral science researchers to look at the problems of prescription pain drug abuse affecting older adults. This problem will only get worse as record numbers of baby boomers approach their sixites. This is a unique population that continues to work beyond 65, where living with pain and decreased mobility is even more pronounced as financially, many cannot afford to retire. Common drugs people seek out for pain are opioids, which are referred to as narcotics and include codeine and morphine, oxycodone (OxyContin), propoxyphene (Darvon), hydrocodone (Vicodin) and hydromorphone (Dilaudid), as well as meperidine (Demerol). Living with chronic pain can create terrible problems with anxiety and general coping. Many people wind up taking further medications known as depressants, which are substances that can slow normal brain function and help with anxiety and sleep disorders. Commonly prescribed medications for these purposes include barbiturates, such as mephobarbital (Mebaral) and pentobarbital sodium (Nembutal), which are used to treat anxiety, tension, and sleep disorders. Benzodiazepines, such as diazepam (Valium), chlordiazepoxide HCl (Librium) and alprazolam (Xanax) are frequently prescribed to treat anxiety, acute stress reactions and panic attacks; the more sedating benzodiazepines, such as triazolam (Halcion) and estazolam (ProSom) can be prescribed for short-term treatment of sleep disorders.

When you look at the number of chemicals used to treat severe chronic pain it becomes clear that a book such as this one is a necessary contribution to anyone's personal health library.

The need for alternative information on injury management has been magnified as several older celebrities have gone on record about their pain medication addictions—addictions that began with debilitating pain from back injuries. Jerry Lewis and Elizabeth Taylor have long been public with their struggles with injury pain. And in the more recent case of Rush Limbaugh's pain medication addiction, he admitted in a press release that severe pain in his lower back and neck due to herniated discs started his addiction.

In national surveys physicians find it difficult to discuss prescription drug addiction with their patients, yet information on alternatives to pain management is not commonly available.

Our intent with this book is to fill a noticeable gap in the injury recovery market. It is intended as a complementary text, and we encourage you to discuss its contents with your doctors; indeed, with anyone suffering from chronic pain due to injury.

M. Sara Rosenthal, Ph.D.
Publisher, Your Health Press

FOREWORD

Healing Injuries the Natural Way is especially close to my heart and philosophy of healing. As I have relayed in past interviews and works, when I was 21, in 1966, I was in Vietnam, and was exposed to Agent Orange on many occasions. As a result, I suffer from peripheral neuropathy, which means "body-wide nerve disease." Both of my legs have a limp, and I have limited use of my arms and hands. When the allopathic system of medicine—the conventional medical model in North America—failed to offer me solutions, I became a pioneer in the alternative nutrition movement and learned to help myself. To my knowledge, I am the longest-known survivor with Agent-Orange induced peripheral neuropathy. The average lifespan after exposure to Agent Orange is five years after deterioration begins—and for me it has been 18 years. Agent Orange has to be in the body for 20 years before it begins to cause deterioration. In 1970, I learned about the lymph system, and how I could clean it to lose weight and clear up other conditions. That effort, it turns out, wound up saving my life. I published my own nutritional healing "belief system" in my first book, *Fit for Life*, and it remains one of the best-selling health books of all time.

Clearly, the healthcare consumer has spoken: this consumer is no longer satisfied with the "take a pill" medical model. Most of us straddle a variety of healing systems and healing "methodologies." We are living amidst an epidemic of bodily injury, due to both aging, and a North American standard of living that breeds inactivity and ill-health. Osteoporosis is at an all time high (in spite of the vast quantities of dairy we consume) as is obesity. People lack the strength and mobility they ought to have, considering the abundance of North American culture.

As a pioneering critic of the current medical model and the nutritional standards already in place, I appreciate the merging of Michelle's personal and professional experiences, which result in this "one-stop" guide to natural healing for people recovering from injuries of all kinds. Michelle has not only "been there" as a survivor of a car accident, but is also a doctor of natural medicine and acupuncture. Michelle has mined the annals of the natural/alternative healing movement, and brings to you a wealth of practical information.

If I can be victorious over Agent Orange, the most toxic man-made chemical ever concocted, you can heal your own injuries, too, aided by the information and techniques in this book.

HarveyDiamond
Best-Selling Author, *Fit For Life* series

INTRODUCTION

If you have been injured and want to overcome your injuries using natural and holistic means, you have come to the right place. This book provides a unique approach to healing various types of bone, soft tissue, and joint injuries based on over a decade of research I have conducted and my personal experience as a Doctor of Acupuncture, Holistic Nutritionist, Biofeedback Therapist, Reiki Master, and Energy Medicine Practitioner.

Unlike most books that offer temporary band-aid-type solutions in the form of over-the-counter (OTC) or prescription pain medications to alleviate pain and inflammation but do nothing to aid healing, *Healing Injuries the Natural Way* offers you an eight-week program that goes to the source of your injuries to help them heal. Using this revolutionary program, you will be providing your body with powerful nutrients it needs to heal and herbs and foods that lessen pain and inflammation. It will teach you how to avoid foods that worsen injuries (yes, foods are some of the worst culprits to stall or inhibit healing), strengthen and stretch the injured areas to enable them to properly heal, and incorporate holistic therapies, which accelerate healing and lessen discomfort along the way.

Healing Injuries the Natural Way is based on my own experience in recovering from severe car accident injuries and my research and knowledge as a health professional who combines Eastern and Western methods of healing.

Ten years ago, I suffered serious injuries in a car accident. The soft tissue in my body was severely damaged. I also experienced a spinal contusion that left my left arm partially paralyzed. For years afterward, I suffered from daily migraines that never seemed to dissipate. I was left with brain inflammation and severe neck and back pain that led to arthritis. I fractured my knee and soon after the accident began to suffer with fibromyalgia, a disorder that left me with whole body aches and pains. Throughout, I suffered from severe and disabling fatigue that was later diagnosed as chronic fatigue syndrome.

For seven years I suffered from relentless migraines and excruciating back and neck pain until I honed in on some of the possible factors that were at play. My injuries were affected by just about everything I did and consumed, leaving me in a state of constant pain and thereby preventing me from getting to the sources of the aggravation. Initially, I tried strong medications that did little to resolve my pain and nothing to help me address the problem. I tried lengthy bouts of physiotherapy, which provided minor improvements in my knee but unfortunately damaged my spine further. A chiropractor (the fourth or fifth I had been to since the accident) finally helped provide some relief, enough that I was able to determine foods and activities that were worsening the injuries.

Finally, my healing journey to overcome the car accident injuries began. After regular chiropractic visits and exercises at home, my migraines lessened. The pain in my body also improved for the first time in years. I finally felt human again. I was reclaiming my life.

Once the pain lessened somewhat, I was able to research options to improve my healing even further. I learned about herbs, foods, juices, vitamins and minerals, along with therapies to help heal my injuries. I went back to school to obtain my Doctorate degree in Acupuncture and later my Doctor of Natural Medicine designation. I also studied various types of energy medicine around the world.

Along the way, I learned about the body's incredible innate wisdom in healing injuries. I also learned that many of the foods we eat, postures we hold, and approaches to life inhibit healing.

While I found a few books on the topic of injuries, I was disappointed with the approaches presented and found little relief by following their programs. I decided to write *Healing Injuries the Natural Way* to help others overcome the disabling effects of injuries, whether they are accident or sports related, to prevent them from suffering needlessly for so many years the way I did. In fact, this book is intended for anyone, male or female, young or not so young, who is suffering from an injury, whatever the injury and its cause.

Healing Injuries the Natural Way combines my personal experience and experimentation, research, and work with clients to offer you an approach to healing that lessens your pain, reduces inflammation, accelerates healing, and improves the quality of your life. I am eternally grateful for the assistance I received on my healing journey and I hope to offer the same to you.

In no way is this book a thorough treatise on each type of injury. To do so would necessitate a lengthy series of books, most of which would take the form of physiology and pathology textbooks. Other books serve that purpose so I won't attempt to duplicate their efforts.

This book will therefore not explain all the different possible types of injuries, nor will it provide for the most part medical names for the injuries discussed. If you want to know about an injury not mentioned in the book or more about one that is mentioned, I recommend you do your own research. The focus of *Healing Injuries the Natural Way* will be to do exactly what the title suggests: it will describe essential insights into healing, whether you're looking to heal bones, muscles, joints, or soft body tissues.

Much of the approach to healing discussed in the book is similar regardless of the type of injury sustained. You will learn about foods that heal and foods that aggravate injuries, herbal healing, nutritional supplementation, aromatherapy, homeopathy and other holistic therapies that help with pain, inflammation, and injuries. You will learn some basic exercises to strengthen and stretch (when appropriate). However, I highly recommend you consult a qualified healthcare specialist who is familiar with your particular injury before embarking on an exercise program.

You will also learn acupressure techniques to balance your body's energies while improving both symptoms and overall healing.

My purpose in writing this book is to empower you to take charge of your body and its healing, and to teach you some of the many natural approaches to healing—approaches that differ from the pharmaceutical model. I will not be recommending prescription medications in this book; please consult a qualified family physician for that information.

While it can be easy to run to a family doctor for every problem that arises, I believe that once you have: a) ruled out serious conditions or b) achieved a diagnosis; it is critical to remember that it is *your* body. You have the power to make choices that will either hinder or help your success with healing. Your body is trying every second and every millisecond to heal. It has an innate intelligence that coordinates literally billions of functions every second, most of which occur on a subconscious level. The body simply does what it needs to do, provided it has all the raw materials to enable it to do so.

That is where *Healing Injuries the Natural Way* comes in. It will help you understand what your body needs so it can do its best healing. You will learn how to provide your body with the best possible raw materials so that it can heal faster and more completely.

You will also learn about the latest research on pain and how you can use the information for powerful healing and pain reduction. I have incorporated much of this insight into my Eight-Week Injury-Healing Program to help you take advantage of this wealth of research.

I wish you tremendous success with overcoming your injuries. It is my hope that this book inspires you to heal yourself and then to compassionately share your knowledge and success with others to help them with their healing.

Yours in healing,

Michelle Schoffro Cook

1
WHEN BONES BRUISE, FRACTURE OR BREAK

Because the bones in our bodies are not visible to us, instead of valuing the important role they play in our overall health we tend to take them for granted, until we succumb to an injury.

Bones as Key Players in Our Overall Health

Bones are our support system. They give our bodies structure. When they fracture or break we become intimately aware of how important they are and the vital role they play in maintaining our body's balance, posture and overall health. We often think of bones as being non-living, concrete-like substances that have little to do other than support us. This is a myth.

Bones are integral to the overall health of our bodies in many ways. We take their many functions for granted until we fracture or break a bone and feel the excruciating pain as our bodies alert us immediately to the injury.

Bones are alive—as much as any other tissue in our body. They're made up of living cells that are almost 50 percent water. All of our blood cells are manufactured in the marrow of our bones. Bones are just as important to every function of the body as they are to the structural make-up of the body. Bones are integral to our heart, lungs, kidneys, muscles, and everything else since our bodies need a constant supply of healthy blood. Every single cell in our bodies depends upon our bones to keep them alive. Some bones, like the skull and ribs, protect the delicate organs beneath them. Also, bones act as a type of holding place for essential chemical elements for the body. Excess nutrients are either excreted in the urine or are deposited on the bones. When the body has a shortage of a particular nutrient elsewhere, it can draw upon the bones to replenish its stores and be used where it is needed most.

Bones also help maintain our body's hormonal balance. Hormonal messengers are sent to the bones when our cells need help from them. Our bones store many minerals to enable the body to draw upon them if, or when, they're needed to help the body function at its peak.

Bones are made up of a living protein network to which minerals attach themselves. Not all of these minerals are essential to bone building. According to Dr. Bernard Jensen, author of *Dr. Jensen's Guide to Body Chemistry & Nutrition*, there are more than two-dozen elements in bones that have no known function (at least at this time in our understanding of the body). Toxic elements such as lead, cadmium, mercury, polonium, and radium are often found in bones as well. When they are stabilized with other nutrients, these toxins appear to do no harm in small quantities.

The minerals calcium, phosphorus, and magnesium are found in the bones in large quantities. On average, our bones contain about 1.4 kilograms of calcium, 680 mg of phosphorus, and 25 mg of magnesium. Almost 99 percent of the body's calcium is found in the bones.

Bones, Them Bones, Them Dry Bones

Bones are constantly being rebuilt by cells called osteoblasts and broken down by cells called osteoclasts. Bone becomes weak when the destruction of bone exceeds the rate of rebuilding.

Similar to a bank that lends money, bones often lend minerals to other parts of the body when they're needed for maintaining our health. If we're always replenishing the minerals in the bones there is no problem; however if our bodies keep borrowing minerals without ever replacing them in the bones, our bones can become fragile and weak. The body appears to have a priority system in place where it borrows from the bones (a lower priority) to ensure higher-priority parts of the body (such as the central nervous system) receive all the nutrients they need.

If you always borrowed money and never paid it back, you would develop credit problems and would become a burden to the bank (or worse). Similarly, if your body is always borrowing minerals from your bones, it leaves the bones susceptible to different kinds of injuries.

Types of Bone Injuries

Bones can be injured in many different ways, including bruising, breaking and fracturing, and these injuries can occur in different parts of the skeletal system.

Breaks and Fractures

Fractures are hairline cracks that form on the surface of the bone. Breaks occur when the bone splits into more than one piece. Bones can fracture or break due to a severe injury or from a lesser injury if the bone mass is weakened due to mineral depletion. A fracture produces swelling and pain that is aggravated by movement. An "avulsion" fracture occurs when a muscle contracts so strongly that it actually pulls away the bone where the tendon is attached.

Most fractures and breaks require the injured area to be immobilized to allow proper healing. Usually this is done with a cast. Some fractures require surgery to pin the pieces of bone together.

Treatment for Common Bone Injuries

It would be impossible to describe treatment options for every kind of bone injury since there are more than 200 bones in the body and therefore many possible types of breaks or fractures. Fortunately, the treatment for most bone injuries is quite similar.

If you've experienced a head injury, or suspect a broken or fractured bone elsewhere in the body, it is important to begin by seeking appropriate medical attention. If you suspect a fracture or broken bone, you should go to the nearest hospital emergency room for treatment. Do not attempt to eat or drink anything. Gently apply an ice pack for short periods to the affected area. The ice pack should be wrapped in cloth before applying it to the skin to prevent ice burns. If the eye is injured, never leave the ice pack on for longer than five minutes as the cold can cause further eye damage. If you suspect a fractured jaw, it can be supported using a scarf or cloth below the jaw and tied over the head, neither too tight nor too loose.

The following list includes many of the common sites for fractures or bone breaks. While the medical treatment may differ from one injury to another, depending on the severity or area that needs immobilization, the rebuilding of bones is basically the same, regardless of the location.

Head and Face Injuries

Andrew Pallas describes the following as signs of skull fractures in his book *Beating Sports Injuries*:

- blood or a clearish-yellow fluid leaking from the ears, eyes or nose;
- bruising around the eyes or behind the ear.

Head injuries can occasionally cause bleeding, which can be serious if it involves the brain. Signs of this type of problem may not become apparent immediately. It is important to pay attention to any unusual symptoms that arise and report them to your physician. If you develop a headache, vomiting, abnormally slow pulse and breathing, or drastic mood changes, be sure to report these problems to your doctor.

Pallas suggests that fractures of the facial bones can cause numerous symptoms, including:

- double vision;
- cheek numbness;
- painful eye movement;
- the pupils of the eyes appearing to be at different heights.

If the fracture has occurred in the jaw, some of the symptoms include:

- pain upon opening the mouth or clenching teeth;
- misaligned teeth when the mouth is closed.

A broken or fractured nose isn't usually serious but be sure to visit a hospital should the nose need to be reset. To control bleeding, lean your head forward.

A serious blow to the eyes can cause something called a "blow-out" fracture, whereby bones in the eye socket become damaged. If you suffer a blow to the eyes or if your vision becomes blurry after an eye injury, visit a hospital immediately.

Neck Injuries

Neck injuries have a wide range of consequences, from minor to life threatening. Injuries to the neck are common; however, serious ones are not. Be careful how you treat someone who may have suffered a fractured neck. Typically, this type of injury can be detected because a person may not be able to move one or more of their limbs, or may be unable to feel you touching their limbs. If a person is unconscious, assume there may be serious injuries, unless you know otherwise. Do not move a person who may have suffered a neck fracture unless they've stopped breathing (so CPR can be performed) or if their surroundings pose a serious threat (such as a burning car or house). If you must move the injured party, try under all circumstances to keep the person's head in line with his or her body. In the case of neck injuries, the site of the pain or numbness may differ from the actual injury site.

Collarbone Injuries

Collarbone fractures or breaks are common injuries, although that makes them no less painful to the many people who suffer from them. Usually this kind of injury is indicated by pain and swelling in the collarbone area and a change in the normal line of the bone.

Arm Injuries

Fractures or broken bones in the arm usually cause severe pain and swelling along with a possible change to the normal shape of the bones. Most injuries to the bones in the arm heal with a cast, although more complex injuries may require surgery.

Wrist and Hand Injuries

Fractures of the wrist are commonly caused by a fall directly onto the hand. Fractures to the bones of the forearm (the radius and ulna) cause pain and swelling, similar to other fractures or breaks. Injuries to the small bones of the wrist, the carpals, cause similar symptoms. Because fractures to one of these bones, known as the scaphoid, cause no visible deformity and may not appear on X-rays, this injury is often misdiagnosed as a sprained wrist. If a so-called "sprained wrist" does not heal after two weeks, you may wish to re-visit your doctor for another examination. Partial immobilization of the affected area is required for up to six months, depending on the severity of the injury. For fractures or broken fingers, treatment usually entails a finger immobilizer, which is typically a padded aluminum strip held in place at the wrist.

Spinal Injuries

Injuries to the spine are typically quite serious. Fractures or broken bones in the spine can result in partial or complete paralysis. Because of the serious nature of this type of injury it is critical to seek medical assistance immediately. Do not move a person who you suspect has suffered a spinal injury, unless the person has stopped breathing or the surrounding situation poses a threat to the person. In that case, carefully move the person onto his or her back to perform CPR. Otherwise, seek medical assistance.

One of the main symptoms of fractures or breaks to the vertebrae of the spine is the inability to move one or more limbs, or to feel someone touching the limbs or torso.

Rib Injuries

Blows to the chest can result in rib fractures or breaks. Fractures or broken bones in this area produce pain, tenderness, and sometimes swelling over the injury site. Coughing, sneezing, deep breathing, or pressure on the chest may aggravate pain. If breathlessness develops, get to a hospital immediately, as broken ribs can cause lung damage.

Hip Injuries

Fractures of the hips are most commonly the result of weakened bones from osteoporosis. In fact, among people suffering from osteoporosis, hip fractures are the most common injury. As they are potentially serious, seek medical attention immediately if you suspect a hip fracture.

Leg Injuries

Broken or fractured legs are usually the result of a severe trauma, such as a car accident. As with other types of fractures or breaks, there is usually severe swelling and extreme pain that prevents movement. The leg will normally be placed in a cast to immobilize it, thereby preventing further damage and allowing the bones to heal.

Knee fractures have similar symptoms but may also involve deformity of the joint. This type of injury is usually caused by a fall onto the knee or a severe blow to the knee. It involves immobilizing to aid healing.

Fractures or breaks in the lower leg can affect one or both of the bones (tibia and fibula). Acute fractures in this area are usually traumatic in origin. They involve severe pain and swelling. Chronic fractures often entail ongoing stress to the bones. Both types of fractures involve immobilization. Some involve surgically implanted pins or wire to stabilize the bones.

Foot/Ankle Injuries

Fractures to the ankles are common. A person suffering from this type of injury typically cannot stand or put weight on the foot due to the tremendous amount of pain. Swelling accompanies this type of injury. Treatment varies depending on the exact location of the fracture and the severity.

The Truth about Osteoporosis

While osteoporosis is not a bone injury in the strictest sense, it is the cause of many bone injuries. According to Harvey Diamond in his book, *The Fit for Life Solution*, osteoporosis currently affects more than 25 million elderly Americans, of whom 80 percent are women. These elderly people currently suffer from 1.3 million fractures every year. In the U.S., more than 20,000 people die every year as a result of hip fractures alone.

For that reason, I feel a book about healing injuries would be incomplete without some discussion of this serious disease. As bones are depleted of their mineral deposits they become more fragile, resulting in the risk of breakages and fractures. Hip fractures are especially common in people with osteoporosis.

As most people already know, osteoporosis is the result of porous bones that are weakened by large withdrawals of minerals, including calcium, over long periods of time. But, there is much more to this disease than a calcium deficiency. In fact, the number of myths surrounding osteoporosis astounds me. Sufferers of this serious illness cannot afford to be fed misinformation, yet it continues, in large part due to corporations that stand to lose large amounts of money if the truth becomes common knowledge, and the media whose advertising budgets are padded by those corporations. Here are the five main myths about osteoporosis.

Myth 1: Osteoporosis Is Just a Calcium-Deficiency Disease

In actual fact, many nutrients and substances are required to prevent bone loss and to strengthen bones. According to Dr. Jensen, they include:

- boron
- calcium
- manganese
- magnesium
- phosphorus
- potassium
- silica
- zinc
- Vitamin A
- Vitamins B: Vitamin B-9 (folic acid), Vitamin B-6, and Vitamin B-12
- Vitamin C
- Vitamin D3 (cholecalciferol)

- Vitamin K
- betaine hydrochloric acid
- glucosamine sulphate
- ipiflavone (7-isopropoxy-isoflavone)

Calcium is a critical mineral in the development of strong bones, but so are the other nutrients and substances I just listed. The body cannot absorb calcium if there isn't enough magnesium and Vitamin D present for assimilation. Also, calcium does not absorb well in a body whose blood is acidic (more on this later).

Bones also require adequate levels of the mineral phosphorus, which in turn is dependent on magnesium. So, as you may have already guessed, the body requires calcium, phosphorus, and magnesium along with Vitamin D in adequate quantities. And, this synergistic relationship continues.

The hormones estrogen and testosterone also help the body assimilate calcium as well. Both men and women have these hormones, although estrogen levels tend to be higher in women while testosterone levels tend to be higher in men. This isn't always the case, however. Both hormones are critical to proper calcium absorption in the bones.

Boron is a trace mineral that increases absorption and utilization of calcium and helps strengthen bones. Jensen cites research that shows boron boosts blood levels of estrogen and other hormones that prevent calcium loss and demineralization of bones. According to Jean Carper, author of *Food: Your Miracle Medicine*, "in other words, boron acts as a mild 'estrogen replacement therapy'" in post-menopausal women who are deficient in this hormone.

The body requires boron to retain calcium, according to research at the U.S. Department of Agriculture's Human Nutrition Research Center in North Dakota. Dr. Forrest H. Nielsen found that post-menopausal women on low-boron diets were more likely to displace calcium and magnesium from their bodies. When they received three mg of boron per day, their calcium losses dropped by 40 percent. Dr. Nielsen believes boron works by boosting natural steroids manufactured by the body in the blood. It increases levels of estrogen and estradiol 17B to double, thereby reaching the same levels as women on pharmaceutical-based estrogen replacement therapy.

The average person in North America gets only half the amount of boron found in the study to be effective at preventing bone demineralization. Dr. Nielsen believes that insufficient consumption of boron could explain why people who consume large quantities of calcium still get osteoporosis. It could also explain why vegetarians typically are less likely to get osteoporosis since they typically eat higher amounts of the fruits and vegetables high in boron.

Boron is found in greatest concentrations in fruits, especially pears, grapes, raisins, dates, peaches, and apples; legumes, especially soybeans; nuts, especially hazelnuts and almonds; and in honey.

Manganese is another mineral that is crucial to proper bone formation and plays a critical role in bone strengthening. Jensen also discusses the following study on manganese's role in bone disorders. Dr. Jeanne Freeland-Graves, Professor of Nutrition at the University of Texas at Austin, found that animals deficient in manganese develop severe osteoporosis. She believes the same is true of people. She found that women with osteoporosis had one-third less manganese in their blood than healthy women. When she administered manganese to the women with osteoporosis, she found their bodies absorbed twice the amount as the healthy women, which suggests that their bodies needed it. Pineapple is high in manganese in a form that is easily digested and absorbed by the body. Other foods that contain manganese include nuts, cereals like oatmeal, tea, spinach, beans, and whole grains.

There are others:

- Magnesium is a mineral that helps the body absorb and metabolize calcium.
- Phosphorus is a mineral that plays a role in bone mineralization and the synthesis of collagen (a glue-like protein that helps hold everything together).
- Potassium is another mineral that enhances calcium absorption.
- Silica is required for the formation of collagen in bone. It also aids with the healing of bone fractures.
- Zinc is a critical mineral for normal bone development and growth and works synergistically with calcium.
- Vitamin A is an essential nutrient that aids in the formation of bones and teeth.
- Vitamin B9 (folic acid), Vitamins B-6 and B-12 are helpful in protecting the body from a build-up of homocysteine (a protein byproduct that interferes with collagen formation necessary for bone development and increases the risk of aging-related diseases).
- Vitamin C is essential to produce adequate levels of collagen and in the formation of bones.

- Vitamin D3 (cholecalciferol) is a vitamin that helps draw calcium from the blood into the bones, thereby stimulating the absorption of calcium from supplements and the diet to form stronger bones.
- Vitamin K is required for the production of osteocalcin (a bone protein), which provides structure to bone tissue. It is critical to bone repair. Without it, bones become fragile and break easily.
- Betaine hydrochloric acid (or betaine hydrochloride) increases the stomach acid to ensure adequate absorption of minerals.
- Glucosamine sulfate is an amino sugar that plays a critical role in the formation of bone.
- Ipiflavone (7-isopropoxy-isoflavone) is a nutrient that inhibits the loss of bone cells. In conjunction with calcium, Vitamin D and other nutrients, it increases bone mineral density, stimulates bone cells, and enhances calcium absorption.

Myth 2: Osteoporosis Can Be Helped or Prevented by Eating More Dairy Products

Many natural health practitioners, myself included, strongly disagree with this statement. While the various dairy-promotion agencies suggest otherwise, my colleagues counter that the truth is, the higher the intake of dairy products, the greater the risk of developing osteoporotic bones.

Here is the reasoning behind this debate: just because a food contains calcium, it does not mean your body will absorb calcium. The U.S. and Canada have two of the highest rates of osteoporosis in the world, which is ironic considering that North Americans drink more milk, eat more cheese, ice cream, and yogurt, and pop more calcium supplements than most other countries in the world.

Yes, it is true that dairy products are some of the highest sources of calcium. However, the body must digest, utilize, and absorb this calcium. There are many biochemical problems in the way in which dairy products are broken down by the body. What many so-called "experts" are not considering is some basic biochemistry with respect to the way in which dairy products are USED by the body, or more accurately, NOT USED by the body.

While dairy foods may be high in calcium when studied in a laboratory, the body does not offer the same conditions as a laboratory. Conversely, the conditions of the body cannot be simulated in a laboratory. In addition, because each person is different, the laboratory cannot account for biochemical individuality.

Based on the research presented in Harvey Diamond's book, *The Fit for Life Solution*, we know that dairy products are apparently not required to combat osteoporosis or develop strong bones. According to the University of Washignton's Women's Health National Center of Excellence, the average calcium intake among Asian women is about half that of Caucasian women in the West, yet the osteoporosis rates are about the same. Asian women have lower hip fracture rates, but more spinal fractures. However, more recent data from the far East is showing that hip fractures in Asian women are sharply increasing. I believe this increase is the result of Western-type dietary influences. Dairy products are extremely acid forming in the body. Acidic blood requires, you guessed it, CALCIUM pulled from the bones to neutralize all that acid in the blood. Nationally renowned microbiologist and nutritionist, Robert O. Young, Ph.D., D.Sc, and Shelley Redford Young state in their recent book, *The pH Miracle: Balance Your Diet, Reclaim Your Health*, "Overacidification of body fluids and tissues underlies *all* disease, and general 'dis-ease' as well." They add: "No matter how many times you were told by teachers and parents to drink your milk, and cute milk moustache ads notwith-standing, the idea that dairy products are healthy is pure hype—a cultural myth. Even if cows lived in some kind of bovine utopia and produced the perfect milk, let's face it: It simply isn't a human food. It is designed for baby cows, whose requirements are far different from those of humans...No other animal species drinks milk beyond infancy: and certainly not from a species outside their own!" (77).

Harvey Diamond, nutrition expert and author of *Fit for Life*, the world's best-selling health book of all time, says: "In the same way that we have been conditioned to think of meat whenever the word 'protein' is mentioned, we have also been taught to believe that dairy products are the finest source of calcium, and the best means by which to prevent osteoporosis. That is precisely what the dairy industry, which makes bil-lions of dollars selling dairy products, wants you to believe, and once again is patently untrue."

Diamond adds: "It is a well-established fact that the high protein content of meat and dairy products turns the blood acidic, which draws calcium out of the bones. This causes the body to lose or excrete more calcium than it takes in. The deficit must be made up from the body's cal-cium reserve, primarily the bones resulting in osteoporosis. This isn't new information. It has been known since 1920 that protein from meat (and dairy-product) consumption causes a net loss of calcium."

Diamond explains: "The countries of the world that consume the greatest amount of dairy products have the highest incidence of osteoporosis! The countries that consume the lowest amount of dairy products have the lowest incidence of osteoporosis."

The recommendations for getting 1,000 mg or more per day of calcium are based on eating an ultra acidic diet. Acid forming foods require large amounts of calcium to buffer the acid in the blood and tissues.

So, what are the acid forming foods? Well, many of the common foods in the Western diet are acid forming, such as: animal protein, dairy, sugar (and all the myriad sugar substitutes), trans-fats, margarine, white and wheat flour and the resulting pastas, breads, and cereals.

Most vegetables and many fruits (raw) are alkalizing to the body. Many whole grains are predominantly neutral (neither acid nor alkaline) in the body.

Myth 3: Osteoporosis Is Unaffected by Lifestyle

Osteoporosis is primarily a lifestyle disease. Living a sedentary life greatly increases a person's likelihood of suffering from this disease. One of the best ways of preventing osteoporosis is to do significant amounts of bone-building exercise, especially while still under the age of 30. However, all people of all ages require exercise. So, if you missed your bone-building activity prior to age 30, start now. It is only too late if you never start exercising.

Calcium is "coaxed" into the bones with adequate exercise. So, pay no attention to those health programs that tell you to pop some pills and forget exercising. The only way to ensure healthy bones is through adequate exercise.

Some of the best forms of exercise for building bone mass include: weight-lifting, or other weight-bearing activities like brisk walking, jogging, working out on an elliptical trainer, in-line skating, rebounding (on a mini-trampoline) or yoga. After a fracture or break has occurred, however, a person will need to allow adequate resting time before embarking on a gradually increasing, gentle exercise program. Not all forms of activity are possible for all people and will depend on a person's level of health, level of fitness, and the severity and location of the injury.

A lesser-known contributor to osteoporosis is depression. According to a recent report by ABC News, "growing evidence suggests that depression, one of the most common diseases of the brain, is so powerful it can actually erode bones in the body."

In *Food: Your Miracle Medicine*, Jean Carper recounts findings by Dr. Philip Gold, head of the Clinical Neuroendocrinology Branch at the National Institute of Mental Health, who has been conducting research on the link between depression and bone density. He suggests that "if you're a pre-menopausal woman and you've had major depression you have a 25 to 30 percent chance of having lost significant amounts of bone and are at a much higher risk of fracture."

Because depression is like a severe state of stress, it causes blood pressure, heart rate, and hormones to increase to dangerous levels. The excess levels of stress hormones cause the depletion of bone minerals, resulting in a loss of bone density.

Even depression that lasts only a few months can cause significant depletion of bone density for both men and women, although it affects the genders differently. Gold's research shows that men who become depressed lose bone density faster and to a greater extent than women. But, men typically have greater bone density to begin with, making them less at risk for fractures or breaks due to bone density loss.

Based on estimates of researchers at the National Institute of Health, 400,000 American women in their 30s and 40s have brittle bones as a result of depression. According to David Keith's recent article, "Build Stronger Bones Naturally," in *Health 'N Vitality* magazine, here are some of the main factors that accelerate or contribute to loss of bone mass:

- aging;
- nutritional deficiencies;
- lack of physical activity;
- being post-menopausal;
- Caucasian or Asian ancestry;
- smoking;
- high caffeine intake;
- alcohol overuse;
- excessive use of certain medications (antacids, cortisone and other steroids, diuretics, and thyroid hormones);
- a family history of osteoporosis;
- prolonged hormonal/endocrine imbalances;
- being female and over 50;
- a low calcium diet;
- poor digestion (inadequate hydrochloric acid and enzymes);
- small body and bone size;
- a history of dieting;

- hysterectomy;
- a diet high in protein and fat;
- weak adrenal glands; and
- a high sodium diet.

I would add:

- an acidic blood pH.

Myth 4: Osteoporosis Only Affects Women

Women aren't the only ones who get osteoporosis, contrary to popular belief. While it is true that women are the main victims of osteoporosis, this disease is affecting a growing number of men. Currently, 20 percent of all post-menopausal women have acquired osteoporosis.

However, older men account for approximately 30 percent of hip fractures resulting from osteoporosis, according to *Food: Your Miracle Medicine*. Yet, osteoporosis is still more prevalent in women because women tend to have smaller bones (on average). Larger bones simply tolerate calcium-depletion better.

In his article, "Build Stronger Bones Naturally," David Keith suggests that more than two million Canadians are at risk of developing osteoporosis. Current estimates propose that one out of four Canadian women and one in eight Canadian men over the age of 50 will suffer from an osteoporosis-related fracture in their lifetime.

Myth 5: Osteoporosis Can Be Prevented by Taking Calcium Supplements

Popping calcium supplements is insufficient to ward off or heal fractures or broken bones linked to bone demineralization for several reasons.

Not all forms of calcium found in supplements are equally digestible or absorbable by the body. Calcium citrate is necessary for building and maintaining bones. This particular form of calcium is more absorbable than other types. However, this is not the main form of calcium found in most supplements. Typically, calcium absorption depends greatly on the amount of stomach acid a person has. Someone with low stomach acid will likely only absorb four percent of most calcium tablets. Calcium citrate is more absorbable. However, if a person suffers from intestinal dysbiosis, Candida, or other digestive troubles, he or she may still get insufficient calcium from pills.

If a person's blood is acidic, the body will use the calcium to alkalize the blood instead of contributing to bone mass since blood acidity is a dangerous state. Unfortunately, most people's blood is highly acidic due to consumption of highly acidic foods. According to some experts, most people need at least 900 to 1,000 mg of calcium per day. However, that is only the case for a person who eats a highly acidic diet (which is virtually everyone in the Western world). This fact may be your single most important piece of information in preventing and reversing osteoporosis. Getting blood acidity under control is critical to bone health.

Osteoporosis is not an inevitable disease that people must succumb to in their later years. It can be prevented and so can the resulting injuries.

Osteomalacia and Bone Injuries

Osteomalacia, which is another disease related to the loss of calcium, also contributes to greater risk of bone injuries. Instead of bones becoming more brittle as they do with osteoporosis, they become more flexible, resulting in deformities and pain. The main cause of this disease is Vitamin D deficiency. The most effective means to reverse osteomalacia is through short-term use of high dosages of Vitamin D. Because high levels of Vitamin D can cause toxicity in the body, it is important to undertake this type of program with a holistic doctor's supervision. One of the best ways to get adequate amounts of Vitamin D is to get responsible amounts of sun exposure on skin. The sun helps the body create Vitamin D. One of the biggest health scams of our time is sunscreen. Not only is the active ingredient in sunscreen a serious carcinogen (causes cancer), it prevents uptake of Vitamin D. I am not condoning unhealthy amounts of sun exposure. I just believe our fanaticism regarding the sun (something that is essential to life) is costing our bodies, namely our bones.

Vitamin D is not required just to prevent osteomalacia. It is essential for bone health in general. It is also required to heal broken and fractured bones. The best way to get adequate Vitamin D is Mother Nature's way— good old-fashioned responsible sun exposure.

Healing Fractures, Broken Bones, Osteoporosis and Osteomalacia

Whether you've been injured in a car accident, a fall, or while playing a sport, if you have a fractured or broken bone, much of the nutritional approach you take toward healing will be the same. The same is true for healing from osteoporosis or osteomalacia.

How to Build Bone the Natural Way

There are a number of ways you can build bones. In addition to following the Eight-Week Injury-Healing Program outlined in chapter 10, I suggest you take the following steps:

- Choose foods that help build strong bones. Your choices should include: high calcium foods, such as salmon, sardines, oysters, shellfish, blackstrap molasses; dark green leafy vegetables, such as broccoli, kale, and collard greens. (For more information about foods that are high in calcium and that have an alkalizing effect on the body, see chapter 4 "Eating for Healing.")
- Eat foods with high boron content, found in greatest concentration in fruits, especially pears, grapes, raisins, dates, peaches, and apples; legumes, especially soybeans; nuts, especially hazelnuts and almonds; and honey.
- Eat raw nuts and fruits, especially fresh pineapple and/or pineapple juice.
- Eat a sensible diet consisting of large quantities of alkalizing fruits and vegetables and whole grains, as described in the Eight-Week Injury-Healing Program in chapter 10.
- Avoid highly acidic foods, such as dairy products, animal protein, sugar products, foods containing trans-fats or hydrogenated fats, soft drinks, etc.
- Try to get regular, small doses of responsible sun exposure.
- Exercise regularly. Try to get regular amounts of weight-bearing activity such as weight lifting, brisk walking, jogging, rebounding, elliptical training, in-line skating, and yoga.

Dealing with Bone Bruising

A bone bruise is an injury to the periosteum, which is a thin sheath that covers the skeletal system. These types of injuries are common in contact sports and are frequently accompanied by pain, swelling and discoloration in the area of the injury.

The homeopathic treatment of ruta (ruta graveolens) is an effective remedy for bone bruises and connective tissue damage, such as injuries to ligaments and joints. Repetitive strain injuries may also be improved with ruta. Common names for the plant from which ruta is derived are "rue" or "herb of grace." This spindly, yellow-flowering herb is native to dry, sunny regions in the Mediterranean.

If ruta does not improve the symptoms within the first 24 hours, symphytum (symphytum officinale) may be used. This remedy promotes bone healing and is derived from comfrey, a plant also known as knitbone. Both ruta and symphytum can be obtained in pill and ointment form. While all potencies are effective, the lower potencies can typically be taken for a longer period of time.

Dealing with Fractures

A fracture may be indicated by pain and/or shock, inability to move the injured body part, swelling, bruising and deformation of the injured area. The injured area should be immobilized to prevent further damage until medical attention can be obtained. Arnica at mid-range potency can be taken every ten minutes to deal with the initial shock and pain of the fracture. It can then be taken every eight hours for up to four days. This may be followed by symphytum at a low potency every eight hours for two or three weeks.

Aromatherapy

The following is a wonderful combination of essential oils to help heal bones and deal with the pain of broken or fractured bones:

- Blend together pure, undiluted oils of eight drops of birch, along with eight drops each of spruce, fir, and helichrysum and seven drops of clove.
- Massage several drops of this combination into the afflicted area (provided there is no broken skin).

Bruised bones also respond well to just helichrysum, an essential oil, used in the same manner as described above.

2
SOFT TISSUE INJURIES

What exactly are soft tissue injuries? "Soft tissue" is an expression commonly used to refer to the "softer" aspects of the outer body, not including bones and joints. Muscles, tendons, and fascia are examples. Soft tissue injuries are commonplace and range from minor to very serious, depending on the nature of the injury.

Muscles

Muscles are the tissues that enable us to move and stay warm. Muscles are arranged in pairs to enable pulling and pushing types of movement. Whenever one muscle in the pair contracts the other is relaxed, and vice versa. This is the basic premise of movement throughout the body. Millions of muscle cells (also known as fibers) operate together to form muscles. The health of the muscles depends on the quality of nourishment they receive. Well-nourished muscle cells are less likely to develop spasms or cramps that lead to pain.

If you've sustained muscle injuries, it is important to be aware of the tendency many people have to adjust posture into a position that alleviates the pain, but which may weaken the structure and create muscular stress.

Tendons

Tendons connect muscles to the bones they move. Injuries to tendons involve either a tear of some of the fibers or a complete rupture, where the tendon is torn in two. Because tendons require less blood supply than muscles to function, they take more time to heal. If a tendon tears near the surface of the body, bleeding from it may produce bruising.

Chronically weakened tendons can occur anywhere, but especially around joints such as the shoulder, knee, elbow, etc.

Tendonitis is the inflammation of the tendons, which are tough bands of tissue that attach muscle to bone. Because tendons are not elastic, they're more susceptible than muscles to inflammation, even from overuse. The most common areas affected are the hips, knees, shoulders, heels, and elbows.

Activities that require a different range of motion than your usual activities are beneficial to increase the resilience of tendons.

Fascia

The tissue that links all the components of the body together is known as "fascia." It carries nerves, blood, and lymphatic vessels through it. Fascia also helps to distribute the weight of the body during movement.

Nerves

Nerves carry information from the brain to the body and vice versa. They allow you to move because the brain can co-ordinate all movements based on signals from the nerves. Nerves also send the brain information about the muscles and joints. Nerves transmit pain signals so the brain knows there is something wrong in the body and can co-ordinate a healing response.

How to Heal Soft Tissue Injuries

There are many types of soft tissue injuries, depending on the type of tissue involved and the location of the injury. Virtually all soft-tissue injuries respond well to the RICE procedure, which entails:

- rest;
- ice;
- compression (this usually entails bandaging the area, but be sure not to bandage it too tightly as this will limit circulation); and
- elevation (elevate the damaged area slightly to limit bleeding and swelling).

Sometimes pain is felt in an area other than the injured area. Andrew Pallas describes "trigger points" in his book *Beating Sports Injuries*, as tender spots, typically in the muscles that cause symptoms to be displaced to other parts of the body.

Soft Tissue Bruising

One kind of soft tissue injury is bruising to the tissue. The discoloration of the skin surface is linked to the rupture of small blood vessels in the tissues beneath the skin surface. This rupture has caused blood and other fluids to leak into the tissues.

Soft Tissue Injuries in the Head

If you've experienced a blow to the head it is important to see a doctor, particularly if you begin to experience dizziness, nausea or vomiting, mood changes, and especially loss of consciousness. If the eye is injured, the tissue involved may become bruised, producing a "black eye." Use an ice pack wrapped in cloth immediately to help with the swelling. Never use an ice pack on the eye for more than five minutes at a time.

Soft Tissue Injuries in the Neck

Neck strains are very common. They can occur from simply turning your head too quickly. These strains usually involve some amount of tearing of the muscles from being over-stretched. Neck strains are more common if the muscles are inflexible. Place a cloth-wrapped ice pack over the neck initially to help alleviate any swelling.

Another form of injury in the neck involves damage to the nerves, referred to as "trapped nerves." Since all but one nerve in the body travel along the spine, any type of more serious spinal injury, including in the neck, can cause nerve damage or a "pinched nerve" if the space between vertebrae lessens. Excellent forms of therapy for this type of injury include: acupuncture and electro-acupuncture, manual therapies like remedial massage, the cranio-sacral technique, chiropractic treatment and exercise.

Thoracic outlet syndrome is similar to pinched nerves but involves both the nerves and blood vessels to the arm. Similarly, "pins and needles" or numbness may be felt due to the pressure on the nerve(s) or reduced blood flow. If the pressure is severe enough, it can cause the hand to swell. The problem area can lie in the neck, collarbone, ribcage, or muscles. Usually, this type of injury is due to a build-up from poor posture or poor form while performing activities, or from an earlier unchecked injury. Chiropractic treatments, massage, acupuncture, the Alexander technique, the cranio-sacral technique, and other manual or postural therapies are suitable for this type of problem.

Soft Tissue Injuries in the Shoulder

Shoulder pain can be the result of injuries anywhere in the neck, chest, or shoulder area. Rotator cuff injuries involve the muscles and/or tendons that move the shoulder joint and give it stability. Because these muscles and tendons are involved in virtually all shoulder movements, they can easily be damaged. They're vulnerable to overuse injuries as well as traumatic ones.

Injuries of the supraspinatus, infraspinatus, and subscapularis are all shoulder muscle injuries. They typically cause restrictive movement of the arm.

Golfer's Elbow and Tennis Elbow

Known to medical professionals as "medial epicondylitis" and "lateral epicondylitis" respectively, these arm injuries are not confined to the courts or the links. Golfer's elbow culminates in inflammation of the flexor and pronator muscles at the humerus, which is the bone of the upper arm. Tennis elbow occurs when the muscles of the forearm are strained at the point where they attach below the elbow. It can also result from an injury to the tendons on the outside of the elbow.

Tendonitis in the Wrist and Hand

The most common types of soft tissue injuries in the hand and wrist are tendonitis (inflammation of a tendon) or tenosynovitis (inflammation of the sheath of a tendon), mainly resulting from overuse of the area. Symptoms usually involve pain with certain movements (usually the type of movement that caused the problem), and creaking.

Back Injuries

Injuries to the soft tissue of the back are common, primarily due to improper posture during activity or from a sudden, jerking movement. The muscles are the primary area affected. Relaxing the injured muscle helps alleviate pain.

Inflammation 101

When soft tissues are injured they usually become inflamed so it is critical to understand healthy ways to deal with inflammation.

Inflammation is a common symptom of many injuries. Any disorder that ends in "-itis" means there is inflammation involved, for example, bursitis, arthritis, etc. Inflammation is the body's healthy response to infection, tissue damage or both. By sending increased amounts of white blood cells to the injured area, the body is better able to repair any damage. Without the inflammation process, injuries would not heal. Most holistic health practitioners feel that taking anti-inflammatory pharmaceutical drugs in fact masks and hence lessens the chances of proper healing.

Martha Moore, A.H.G., describes numerous causes of inflammation in her book, *Beyond Cortisone*, including:

- physical damage (trauma, wounds, burns, sunburns and radiation);
- chemical substances (including some pharmaceutical drugs);
- microorganisms (bacteria, viruses, and parasites);
- ischemia or death of tissues from lack of oxygen;
- foreign particles; and
- all types of immune system reactions including autoimmune conditions and hypersensitivity reactions, e.g., arthritic conditions.

Depending on the nature of the injury, a person who has sustained any or all of the preceding conditions may be experiencing inflammation.

Your Inflammatory Response

The March/April 1994 edition of the online nutrition journal, *Nutri-Notes* described the "inflammatory response" as the body's internal defense mechanism against injury. It is the body's effort to protect itself by neutralizing and destroying toxins at the site of an injury so that any infection cannot spread to other tissues. The following occurs as part of an "inflammatory response:"

1. Blood vessels dilate, increasing in size and becoming more permeable so that substances normally contained in the blood can travel out into tissues, enabling greater blood flow to the site of an injury. The larger volume of blood at the injured site allows the body to remove toxins and dead cells. Increased permeability allows the white blood cells and clot-forming substances to enter the damaged area. This occurs because the body has released chemicals such as histamine, kinins, and prostaglandins. The increased blood circulation and permeability of small blood vessels (known as capillaries) produces heat, redness, and swelling within minutes of an injury. Pain is the

result of damage to nerves, toxin irritation, and/or pressure from the swelling. Prostaglandins worsen and lengthen the pain attributed to inflammation.

2. Kinins also affect nerve endings and contribute to pain.

3. Bacteria-eating cells known as phagocytes migrate to the area to help ward off infection after the inflammation process has begun. The different types of white blood cells squeeze through the capillaries to reach injured tissues, and another type of immune system cell called neutrophils (storage centers for proteolytic enzymes, which I'll discuss later) clear away any toxic debris.

4. Nutrients that the body has stored are released to be used in the area of the injury. They support the defensive immune system cells and injured cells.

While inflammation is the body's means of dealing with injury to soft tissues, if it remains unchecked for lengthy periods of time, then it can cause serious harm to the body. However, even for short durations, inflammation can cause mobility problems and be linked with pain that is difficult to deal with.

Pharmaceutical vs. Natural Approaches to Inflammation

There are more than 200 potential anti-inflammatory drugs, including non-steroidal anti-inflammatory drugs (NSAIDs), corticosteroids (in the form of cortisone injections, creams, etc.), gold salts, methotrexate, and hydroxychloroquine. However, many people find a natural means is best to control inflammation since this approach also promotes healing and does not involve side effects. As well, natural remedies do not interfere with the body's innate ability to heal and repair injured areas.

NSAIDs

NSAIDs include aspirin, acetaminophen (Tylenol), ibuprofen (Advil), and others. Some of the side effects of these medications include: stomach bleeding and ulcers, gastrointestinal distress (heartburn, nausea, stomach pain, vomiting, diarrhea), headaches, dizziness and/or tinnitus, which is a continuous buzzing or ringing in the ears with no obvious cause (and is one of the most common hearing disorders in adults). Over longer periods of time NSAIDs can cause kidney and liver damage. These medications also appear to accelerate the development of osteoarthritis and increase the rate of joint destruction.

Corticosteroids

Corticosteroids are powerful drugs with powerful side effects. They deplete your body's immune system response, thereby making you more prone to infections of all kinds. In addition, they're harmful to the adrenal glands (the stress glands), and can cause depression, high blood pressure, diabetes, cataracts, blurred vision, severe muscular weakness, ulcers, thinning of the skin, and osteoporosis.

More Strikes Against OTC/Prescription Painkillers

According to Dr. Sherry Rogers, author of *Pain-Free in 6 Weeks*, side effects from OTC and prescription drugs are the third highest cause of death in the U.S. When one considers how many of these drugs are in the category of "analgesics" (pain medications), which include the non-narcotic drugs such as NSAIDs (nonsteroidal anti-inflammatory drugs) or narcotic drugs, such as opioids and opiates, this is significant. The OTC and prescription pain medications that millions of people turn to for relief from pain, inflammation, and other symptoms are not only causing side effects, they may actually worsen or aggravate the health of many people. By Dr. Roger's research, 6,000 people die every year from "simple" non-steroidal anti-inflammatory medications. The side effects of these medications contribute to congestive heart failure, kidney disease, suicidal depression, cataracts, ulcers, macular degeneration, hearing loss, tinnitus, memory loss, fatigue, and liver disease.

Prescription and over-the-counter medications also deplete your body of much-needed vitamins and minerals required for all your body's basic functions. Over-the-counter pain relievers like Aspirin, Advil, Aleve, Tylenol, and the countless others on the market deplete your body of Vitamin C, folic acid (Vitamin B-9), iron, and zinc. These nutrients are needed to keep your immune system strong, heal tissues, maintain cellular integrity, build healthy blood, heal wounds, and nourish skin and hair.

Besides that, OTC and prescription pain medications do not eliminate the underlying causes of the symptoms people take them for; instead, they merely mask them. While that pill may help alleviate a symptom in the short term, in the long term, the medications may be creating other problems. The liver and kidneys must filter every synthetic chemical that enters your body, including medications. Repeated use of these medications can weaken these organs and the body's ability to detoxify. Plus, the cause of the original problem that was covered up by medications may rear its ugly head somewhere down the road in a much nastier form.

Drugs Used for Soft Tissue Injuries and the Nutrients They Deplete

Type of Drug	Name	Nutrients They May Deplete
painkillers	Acetylsalicylic Acid Ibuprofen Indomethacin Naproxen Nabumetone	Vitamin C folic acid (Vitamin B-9) iron zinc
steroids (corticosteroids) Often used for asthma, rheumatoid arthritis, colitis, skin disorders, and immune disorders	Prednisone Hydrocortisone Desamethasone Beclomethasone Triamcinolone	pyridoxine (Vitamin B-6) Vitamin C Vitamin D Vitamin K zinc potassium
antidepressants	Amitriptyline Desipramine Doxepin Imipramine	coenzyme Q-10

Before you stop using any drug, it is important to see your physician. Sudden discontinuation of some prescription medications can cause severe health problems.

And if you're taking any OTC or prescription pain medication, you must consider that they may interrupt the delicate workings of the body and deplete vitamins and minerals that the body requires for proper healing. I listed some of the main nutrients that are depleted by several types of OTC and prescription medications in the table above to help you understand their importance.

Common Nutrients Depleted by Some Drugs

Nutrient	Function
Vitamin B-6 (pyridoxine)	Ensures proper nerve function (a deficiency increases your risk of nervous system disorders like carpal tunnel syndrome) Needed for normal brain function and synthesis of DNA and RNA Aids sodium-potassium balance Prevents depression

	Helps process hormones in the liver
	May lower risk of heart disease (by lowering homocysteine levels)
Vitamin B-9 (folic acid, folate, folacin)	Essential for cellular health (a deficiency can cause abnormal cellular growth)
	Needed to produce red blood cells
	Assists with tissue healing
	Strengthens immunity by aiding in the proper formation and functioning of white blood cells
	Reduces risk of birth defects
	May lower risk of heart disease, cervical and colon cancer and depression
Vitamin C (ascorbic acid)	Essential for proper immune function and wound-healing
	Helps build healthy hair and skin
	Doses of 1,000 mg per day may shorten the duration of colds
	Helps protect the body against pollution
	May reduce high blood pressure and prevent arteriosclerosis
	Required for adrenal gland function
	Powerful antioxidant
Vitamin D	Necessary for the absorption of calcium for bone strength (a deficiency can cause bone thinning and may raise the risk of osteoporosis)
	Protects against muscle weakness
	Regulates heartbeat
	Required for normal growth and development of bones and teeth
Vitamin K (phylloquinone)	A deficiency increases bruising and bleeding
	May lower risk of bone fractures and osteoporosis
	May increase resistance to infection
	Promotes healthy liver function
	Essential for bone formation and repair
Iron	Helps your body build healthy blood
	Essential for enzymes and growth
	Required for a healthy immune system and energy production
Zinc	Essential for proper immune function and wound-healing

	Helps build healthy hair and skin
	Protects liver from chemical damage
	Constituent of insulin and many enzymes
	Important for healthy prostate function
	Required for protein synthesis
Coenzyme Q-10	Necessary for a healthy heart
	Powerful antioxidant
	Aids circulation
	Boosts the immune system
	Increases tissue oxygenation
	Has anti-aging effects

What to Use in Place of NSAIDs

The best-known pain-reliever is aspirin. Aspirin's active ingredient is salicin, which converts to salicylic acid in the stomach. Chemists first synthesized salicylic acid in the nineteenth century. The drug was given its name, which reflected its herbal heritage. The herb, meadowsweet, was called "spirea" at the time. Meadowsweet, along with willow bark, contains a natural version of salicylic acid. Herbalists recommend meadowsweet or willow bark for many of the same symptoms for which doctors suggest aspirin. One benefit is that there are fewer side effects with herbs. Two cups of tea or one to two dropperfuls of the tincture are recommended for pain and inflammation. Meadowsweet appears to be less irritating to the stomach than willowbark.

According to Dr. Krishna C. Srivastava of Odense University in Denmark, ginger is superior to NSAIDs in alleviating pain and inflammation. NSAIDs work on one level, blocking the substances that cause inflammation. Ginger works on at least two mechanisms:

- Ginger blocks the formation of prostaglandins and leukotrienes.
- Ginger has antioxidant properties that actually break down inflammation and acidity in the joints' synovial fluid.

Fibromyalgia Syndrome (FMS)

While fibromyalgia is not directly an injury, it frequently starts after an injury, particularly a severe one, such as resulting from a serious car accident. If you're dealing with fibromyalgia as a result of an injury, keep reading. There is no need to suffer so terribly from the all-over aching attributed to this disorder.

Symptoms of Fibromyalgia

The following basic criteria are used to give a medical diagnosis of fibromyalgia syndrome:

- widespread pain in all four quadrants of the body lasting for at least three months;
- tenderness in at least 11 of the 18 specified tender points;
- generalized aches or stiffness of at least three anatomic sites for at least three months; and
- exclusion of other disorders that are known to cause similar symptoms.

In the May/June 2003 issue of *Herbs for Health*, Karta Purkh Singh Khalsa describes minor diagnostic criteria for fibromyalgia as:

- generalized fatigue;
- chronic headache;
- sleep disturbance;
- neurological and psychological complaints;
- joint swelling;
- numbing or tingling sensations;
- irritable bowel syndrome;
- variations of symptoms in relation to activity, stress and weather changes; and
- temporomandibular joint syndrome (TMJ).

Originally termed fibrositis, fibromyalgia is a prevalent type of rheumatism. As a syndrome, it is a collection of seemingly unconnected symptoms with the main one being unaccountable pain ("myo" means muscle; "algia" means pain) in the muscles.

Currently fibromyalgia affects between two and four percent of Americans, with a ratio of seven to one of the patients affected being women. Next to osteoarthritis, FMS is the second most common form of arthritic disorder. While it is a form of arthritis that also affects the joints, the primary symptom is muscular pain, so I have included it in this chapter.

Fibromyalgia may also involve other seemingly unrelated symptoms including chest pain, headaches, tingling, dizziness, constipation, diarrhea, gas, abdominal pain, water retention, premenstrual syndrome, menstrual cramps, sleep problems, restless legs, irritable bladder and poor memory. Symptoms often worsen after heavy exercise.

While its onset may be mysterious, some researchers believe that for many people it may be caused by a forceful trauma, such as a motor vehicle accident or another injury that damages the central nervous system in an as-yet-unknown way.

Some researchers found that fibromyalgia syndrome sufferers appear to have lower levels of somatomedin C, a hormone produced by the liver in response to growth hormone. Somatomedin C is involved in tissue repair at night and is secreted during the deepest phase of sleep. Says Karta Purkh Singh Khalsa, C.D.-N, R.H.: "When we sleep for about one hour in the dead of night, our muscles relax completely. During this short time, the muscles are able to heal at the deepest level; circulation of blood and lymph reaches the deepest cells. If sleep is disturbed, and the muscle remains the slightest bit tense, this healing is impaired, which begins a cycle of chronic subclinical damage that eventually escalates into the physical and mental symptoms of FMS."

Because the pain can be so disabling to people suffering from fibromyalgia, many people refrain from exercise that seems to worsen symptoms. However, over time, the lack of exercise weakens muscle tone, causing less blood and lymph to flow through the body and worsening symptoms. Exercise, started slowly and built up gradually, often improves symptoms.

Karta Purkh Singh Khalsa cites a 2002 Swedish study of the effect of pool exercise on fibromyalgia sufferers. Study participants over six months found lasting improvements in symptom severity, physical function and social function through regular pool exercise.

Karta Purkh Singh Khalsa recounts research that found a link between allergies and fibromyalgia. In a study presented at a 1996 meeting of the American Association for the Advancement of Science, subjects were given blood tests to determine sensitivity to 340 medications, foods, food additives and environmental chemicals. After four months of eliminating those to which they were found to be allergic, most of the subjects felt significant improvement. After six months, they experienced 50 percent less pain, 40 percent less depression, 50 percent more energy and 30 percent less stiffness. Other symptoms such as headaches improved as well.

Magnesium is one of the most critical nutrients needed by people suffering from fibromyalgia syndrome. Research consistently finds that people diagnosed with this disorder are typically quite deficient in this mineral, which is critical for the production of adenosine triphosphate (ATP), the source of energy in muscles. The therapeutic dose varies from person to person but should be used to bowel tolerance (excess magnesium causes loose stools). For most people this is about 1,500 mg per day. Foods that contain significant amounts of magnesium include dark green vegetables, legumes, seeds and nuts.

Karta Purkh Singh Khalsa also recommends kava, turmeric root, willow bark, ginkgo biloba, coenzyme Q-10, ginger root, cayenne, boswellia gum or Indian frankincense, guggul gum and massage therapy for sufferers of fibromyalgia. These herbs and nutrients are also effective for soft tissue injuries.

Healing Soft Tissue Injuries and Fibromyalgia

Kava (piper methysticum) is an analgesic whose potency ranks between aspirin and morphine. It is a muscle relaxant and sleep aid but does not create the negative morning symptoms linked to tranquillizers. Karta Purkh Singh Khalsa recommends taking kava in an alcohol-based tincture (85 percent alcohol), taking one teaspoon at bedtime and working up to one tablespoon. Because kava has been linked to liver damage, it should be used under the guidance of a healthcare practitioner.

Turmeric (curcuma longa) is the yellowish spice commonly used in Indian food. Its main therapeutic ingredient is curcumin, which has been shown to deplete nerve endings of substance P, a pain neurotransmitter. Research shows that curcumin suppresses pain through a similar mechanism as drugs like COX-1 and COX-2 inhibitors (without the harmful side effects).

For acute episodes, people can take up to four tablespoons of turmeric mixed into water or honey per day. I find the honey-turmeric mixture to be far more palatable than taking turmeric in water or juice. For ongoing concerns, one teaspoon per day is sufficient to lessen pain. Turmeric can also be ingested in capsule form. In that case, choose a standardized extract with 1,500 mg of curcumin content per day.

Willow bark is beneficial for joint pain (see chapter 3).

In a 2002 study using ginkgo biloba and coenzyme Q-10, among patients taking 200 mg of CoQ-10 and 200 mg of ginkgo extract daily for 84 days, 64 percent found improvement from symptoms.

Karta Purkh Singh Khalsa recommends one to ten grams per day of ginger root to increase circulation to muscles.

Cayenne improves circulation and reduces pain. Take up to three 500 mg capsules per day. Be aware that some people find even a single capsule causes a burning sensation in the stomach. You can also use cayenne sprinkled on food (1/4 teaspoon is the equivalent of approximately 400 mg).

Boswellia gum or Indian frankincense (boswellia serrata) lessens pain. Use a standardized 65 percent boswellic acid product, 300 to 1,200 mg per day.

Guggul gum (commiphora mukul) is an Ayurvedic herb used for arthritic diseases. You can take two to ten capsules per day, 600 mg per capsule.

Proteolytic enzymes are also effective in healing soft tissue damage because they help rid the body of toxic materials made up of protein, which are released during inflammation and can contribute to disease. "Proteolytic" means the degradation of proteins. Proteolytic enzymes are released by neutrophils, which are cells produced by the body's immune system to engulf and destroy bacteria and dead particulate matter. They release the proteolytic enzymes when they arrive at the injured location to prevent infection. There are many types of proteolytic enzymes that are capable of assisting with lessening inflammation and healing injured tissue. Some of these enzymes have been used topically (on the skin) while others have been used internally with excellent results. In one study, the enzyme trypsin increased the ability of the skin to form new cells when applied to the area. Bromelain, another enzyme, has powerful therapeutic effects when used to treat inflammation and soft tissue injuries, according to Karta Purkh Singh Khalsa. It also reduces skeletal muscle injury. Pineapple (raw, not canned or cooked) contains plentiful amounts of bromelain.

Avoiding Soft Tissue Injuries

The first step you can take is to avoid situations that can lead to soft tissue injury, pain and spasms. Here are some suggestions, taken from an informational flyer, entitled, "Avoiding Injury, Spasms, and Pain" published by Advanced Nutrition Publications, Inc.

1. Take care to achieve and maintain your body's optimal biomechanical function, focusing on accurate bone alignment and proper joint movement.

2. Nourish your various tissues (cartilage, ligaments, tendons, and muscles) with nutrients that help support their ability to heal and prolong their health and vitality.

3. Exercise regularly, even if it involves only a simple range of motion. Movement is essential to accomplish the delivery of nutrients to and the removal of waste products from the cells found in cartilage.

4. Reduce stress as much as possible. Adequate rest following exercise may help promote thorough delivery of nourishment to the cells of the connective tissues.

Foods and Nutrients that Fight Pain and Inflammation

Inflammation is characterized by redness, pain, heat, swelling, and restrictive movement. The healing process that occurs after inflammation places a tremendous demand on the body's store of nutrients, so it is critical to eat well to replenish the supply. Chapter 4 includes a Healing Foods Pyramid diagram and a chart listing healing foods by category, including the top 20 anti-inflammatory and anti-pain foods that are more effective than most OTC and prescription pain medications, the top ten anti-inflammatory and anti-pain spices, many of which are more effective than most OTC and prescription pain medications, the top calcium-rich foods that alkalize the body and foods that contain natural aspirin.

Foods to Alkalize Your Body

While there are many nutrients that aid in the healing of injuries, healthy muscles require lots of calcium and magnesium, which alkalize the body. Calcium aids in the healing of inflamed tissues while magnesium helps decreases swelling. To learn the top calcium-rich foods that alkalize the body, see the Healing Foods Chart in chapter 4. Excellent food sources that are rich in magnesium include: dried figs, seafood, barley, oats, brown rice, rye flour, cocoa, cashews, almonds, brazil nuts, pecans, hazelnuts, walnuts, soybeans, soy flour, most beans and peas, beet greens, chard, spinach, collards, and most types of seaweed.

Using Homeopathy for Soft Tissue Bruises

Arnica (arnica montana) is an effective remedy for contusions. In fact, arnica is the primary remedy for virtually all cases of physical injury due to its ability to relieve pain, reduce inflammation and assist with shock. The plant's healing properties, unlike its many names (leopard's bane, mountain daisy, sneezewort, and mountain tobacco) have been recognized for centuries. Arnica can be taken in doses of 30x or 30c every hour until improvement is noticeable.

Bellis (bellis perrenis), derived from the common daisy (also known as bruisewort, garden daisy or European daisy) is a good remedy to follow arnica. It acts directly on muscle tissues and the blood vessels to promote healing. Bellis has also been used to treat varicose veins and to ease post-surgery pain. Lower dosages (3c, 3x, 6x) are recommended for the treatment of bruises.

Hamamelis (hamamelis virginiana) has also been used to treat varicose veins and bleeding (for instance, bleeding from heavy periods in women). It is also recommended for injuries that result in bruising of the breast tissue. Hamamelis is derived from witch hazel, a plant used by Native Americans for its astringent and anti-inflammatory properties. Ruta and symphytum are also effective in dealing with bruises.

Golfer's Elbow and Tennis Elbow

Arnica is the first choice for muscle injuries. Low- to mid-potencies are suggested every half-hour for the first two hours. Ruta can be taken three to four times a day for several days until the symptoms are noticeably improved. A dosage in the 6x, 30x to 30c range is suggested. Ruta and arnica can both be purchased as an ointment and applied topically to the injury.

Adjunct Healing Therapies for Soft Tissue Injuries

Some of the best healing modalities (in addition to nutrition) to help with soft tissue healing include: acupuncture, homeopathy, chiropractic and gentle manual therapies (provided they do not cause further strain to the injured area), such as cranio-sacral therapy or gentle massage therapy. Also, I suggest the regular use of the acupressure techniques described in chapter 7 to speed healing.

3

DEALING WITH JOINT DAMAGE

J oints are the meeting place of two or more bones. They allow bones to move relative to each other. According to Andrew Pallas in his book, *Beating Sports Injuries*, joints consist of the following four main components:

- ligaments;
- cartilage;
- joint capsule; and
- bursae.

Ligaments

Ligaments are like straps that hold bones together at the joint to add stability. They can become damaged if a force acts too strongly against a joint. For example, ligaments stabilize the joints when bending sideways. If a force pushes the joint too hard in that direction, the ligaments will become damaged. If ligaments are damaged there is usually pain and swelling around the joint. Overstretching the ligaments can cause the joints to become unstable. Chronically weakened ligaments can occur anywhere, but especially around joints, such as the shoulder, knee and elbow.

Cartilage

The ends of bones are covered in cartilage to provide a smooth surface that absorbs some shock. However, damage to the cartilage can make the joints more susceptible to wear. Joints like the knee have additional cartilage to act like washers, filling in gaps between bones that wouldn't otherwise fit exactly.

Joint Capsules

The joint capsule is a type of ligament that forms a bag around the joint to contain a lubricating fluid known as synovial fluid. These keep joints lubricated. The joint capsule can be injured in the same way as other ligaments.

Bursae

These fluid-filled sacs are positioned at key points around certain joints to act as cushions. They separate and pad neighboring tissues. High amounts of stress on a joint can cause the bursa to become inflamed, resulting in swelling. For example, lengthy amounts of time kneeling can cause the bursa at the front of the knee to become sore and swollen. Inflammation of the bursa is known as "bursitis" and can occur in any of the joints of the body. Typically, this type of injury results from overuse of a particular joint.

Many nutrients are imperative to proper healing of cartilage, including Vitamin C and bioflavonoids, zinc, manganese, silica (organic), amino acids, glucosamine sulfate, chondroitin sulfate and others.

Types of Joint Injuries

The main types of joint damage include sprains, dislocations, and cartilage injuries.

Joint Sprains

In a sprain, the ligaments that strengthen a joint become stretched or torn. Typically, partial tears of ligaments heal on their own, but if the ligament is completely torn (ruptured), it usually needs to be surgically repaired or the continuing inflammation can harm other structures of the joint. A severe rupture can cause the joint to become dysfunctional.

Joint Dislocations

When the bones are forced out of their normal positions in a joint, a dislocation is the resulting injury. Usually this occurs because of a serious fall or a contact injury. Shoulder, finger, and thumb joints are the most common sites for this type of injury but it can occur almost anywhere a joint is located. It is imperative that a trained medical professional be seen for this type of injury so that the bone ends can be returned to their proper position. An untrained person trying to force the bone back into its normal position in the socket is likely to cause more damage than good.

Cartilage Injuries

According to James M. Rippe, M.D., author of *The Joint Health Prescription*, the most common type of cartilage injury occurs in the knee. It may occur during contact sports or sports that require sudden twisting movements, like basketball or tennis. Even a sudden, severe jerking motion or a fall can cause a cartilage injury. This type of injury typically requires surgery if the tear is significant enough. During surgery, the fragments of torn cartilage are removed so they do not cause severe inflammation of the joint. If the tear is minor, physiotherapy is usually recommended to strengthen the muscles around the joint.

Risk Factors for Joint Problems

Dr. Rippe suggests that there are many risk factors involved in joint problems, including: age, female gender, being overweight or obese, a previous injury, occupations requiring repetitive motion, muscle weakness and bone problems.

Age

Joint problems increase with age. You cannot change your age, but you can change your "physiological age"—the age that reflects how well you take care of your body.

Female Gender

Women have more joint problems than men, particularly after they reach menopause. The reasons for this phenomenon are not well known.

Overweight and Obesity

If a person is overweight or obese, he or she is at increased risk of joint problems, due to the strain on the joints. Dr. Rippe found that obesity is the leading cause of osteoarthritis in women and the second cause of osteoarthritis in men (next to prior injuries). Extra weight places extra stress on the joints, namely the knees and hips. The stress can cause misalignment of the joints, which further injures them. Weight management is critical to joint health.

Previous Injury

Often a previous injury becomes a weak spot for possible future injuries. While joint injuries cannot be totally prevented, keeping the muscles strong lessens the chances of certain types of joint injuries.

Occupations Requiring Repetitive Motion

Dr. Rippe also cites studies that show people in occupations requiring repetitive squatting or kneeling have an increased likelihood of joint injuries (in the joints that are under stress). It is important to consider adopting preventive measures like wearing kneepads if you must kneel regularly in your profession. People who engage in hobbies that use repetitive motions should take precautionary measures as well. Gardeners, for example, should wear kneepads and be more aware of using proper form when doing routine tasks.

Muscle Weakness

Muscles tend to weaken with age, mostly because people become more sedentary. Muscles and joints work together. The weakness of a muscle can often lead to a joint problem, rather than a joint problem leading to weakened muscles. Stretching and strengthening exercises are essential to proper joint health. Dr. Rippe's research shows that even people in their 80s and 90s can gain function and mobility by incorporating regular stretching and strengthening exercises into their daily routine.

Bone Problems and Joints

Various bone injuries and disorders, including osteoporosis, can lead to joint problems. If you haven't already read chapter 1, I highly recommend going back to that chapter to learn about improving bone health.

Symptoms of Unhealthy Joints

The most obvious symptom of unhealthy joints is pain. Other symptoms include morning joint stiffness, buckling or instability, diminished function (limited range of motion) of the joint, enlargement of the bones around the joint, tenderness when the joint is touched, heat or excess fluid in the joint and deformity.

The Role of Fatty Acids in Joint Health

Injuries can damage cartilage cells, which then release fatty acids that are changed by enzymes into substances that cause pain. This is the body's warning signal to get your attention to the need for healing. Attaining sufficient amounts of the proper fatty acids in one's diet can aid with cartilage healing and reduce pain in several different ways. Replenishing the body's supply of fatty acids is critical to the proper healing of cartilage. In addition, certain dietary fatty acids may serve to reduce the excessive production of the inflammation and pain-causing substances. Dietary fatty acids also lead to production of other substances that alleviate pain. Some of the main types of oils that can assist with cartilage healing include: evening primrose oil, borage oil, flax oil, and fish oils. Consumption or supplementation of these oils is critical to effective healing.

How to Maintain Healthy Joints and Heal Injuries

1. Keep active and exercise regularly. For example, walking regularly can be very beneficial to the health of your joints. "Use it or lose it!" really does apply to maintaining healthy joints. Your body was meant for movement. A sedentary life simply weakens joints. However, if you recently sustained a joint injury, consult your doctor before embarking on any exercise.

2. Strengthen your muscles. You need some form of strength training to maintain healthy joints and joint alignment. Depending on your level of physical fitness, this does not mean that you need to become a body builder. Even regular strength training with small weights or rubber can be beneficial to healing joint injuries or preventing them altogether.

3. Eat healthily. While I have listed this as number three, it is no less important than the other factors. Proper nutrition helps in weight management and ensures that your body's cells get the building blocks they need to be healthy and create healthy tissues and bones. I have included a nutritional program for overcoming injuries, which you will find in the Eight-Week Injury-Healing Program outlined in chapter 10.

For Neck Joint Injuries

A joint sprain in the neck involves tearing the ligaments that support the neck joints. Symptoms are similar to a neck strain in that movement may be limited and painful. There may also be pain at the back of the head, across the shoulder, or down the arm. You may experience a "pins and needles" sensation or tingling in one or more of these areas. As with a strain, begin with using a cloth-wrapped ice pack on the area, and follow the advice provided for dealing with inflammation.

For Spinal Disk Injuries

One of the causes for injury to the cushioning capacity of the disks in the spine is a weakness of spinal ligaments and tendons. A chronic weakening of ligaments and tendons may contribute to overall structural instability, making a person susceptible to improper bone movement and painful misalignment. Injuries to the disks in the spine can occur in various ways. Some are the result of lifestyle and posture, rather than a sudden traumatic injury. Here are some examples:

- *A herniated disc.* This type of injury occurs from chronic weakening of the outer sheath of the disk, which allows the softer center portion of the disk to bulge through, and press on a spinal nerve, causing pain.
- *A degenerated disc.* Over time the entire structure of the disk has become so weak and thin that it no longer provides the proper separation and shock-absorbing effect between the vertebrae. As a result the vertebrae are susceptible to micro-fractures and bone spurs as well as improper movement, which may lead to painful misalignment.
- *Weakening of spinal ligaments and tendons.* See chapter 2 for more information.

Doctors often refer to disc injuries as "slipped discs," but discs do not slip, so this is misleading. Occasionally, injuries to the discs are the result of traumas, but more commonly, they are the result of long-term misuse or misalignment of the body or lack of use of the muscles of the body.

Spinal injuries are INCREDIBLY COMPLEX. The nature and severity will determine the healing program. Many spinal injuries result in paralysis or partial paralysis and therefore require medical attention. Serious spinal injuries may not improve significantly, particularly if nerves become damaged or severed along the spine.

For Shoulder Injuries

Since shoulder dislocations can be accompanied by fractures, seeking a medical opinion initially is integral to proper treatment. Dislocation between the collarbone and shoulder blade can cause a noticeable bump on the top of the shoulder. Nerves and blood vessels that supply the arm can be pinched with a shoulder dislocation injury, resulting in discomfort in the arm and hand.

The bursa (cushioning of the shoulder joint) can become inflamed in shoulder injuries. This is known as subacromial bursitis. It may result in a spongy swelling on the outside of the shoulder. This situation should be treated with the RICE procedure (rest, ice, compression and elevation).

For Elbow Injuries

Dislocations of the elbow joints are rare but may be the result of an awkward fall onto the elbow. Symptoms of an elbow dislocation include: severe pain, swelling, and joint deformity. Treatment usually involves a splint for a week or two.

Small fragments of bone or cartilage can become lodged in the elbow joint, causing pain and stiffness of the area. Typically, this type of injury is the result of repeated throwing actions. Rest is critical to the healing of this injury.

For Wrist Injuries

A sprained wrist resulting from torn ligaments around the joint may involve pain and reduced movement of the wrist joint. However, any type of joint injury that increases mobility is dangerous because the joint becomes unstable. Usually muscles and/or ligaments are stretched out of shape and people have the tendency to overuse the joint, which slows healing. As with shoulder injuries the RICE procedure is an effective treatment to follow.

For Chest Injuries

The joints of the rib cage can be damaged from injuries. Ribs consist of two parts: a bony part and a cartilage part. Sprains involve the joint between the two parts. These types of injuries can be caused by strain or impact. Typically, pain is worsened by deep breathing or upper body movement. Again, follow the RICE procedure for initial treatment.

For Hip Injuries

One can sustain injury in several locations in the hip area, including the sacroiliac joint, the symphysis pubis or pubic bone, and the hip joint itself.

The sacroiliac joints connect the bones at the rear of the pelvis, at the top of the buttocks. These joints have small movements that are nevertheless important to the proper functioning of the body. Sacroiliac joint sprains can be the result of a fall or other awkward movement. They can be the result of seemingly minor, but unexpected, movements that jar the body. Pain can be anywhere in the buttocks, hips, groin, and the back of the thigh or even the foot. Typically, the joint may need manipulation to return it to a normal position.

Sciatica is pain that radiates from the hip down the leg. It is not truly an injury, but a symptom of a problem. Problems from the sacroiliac joint can be the culprit. Other possibilities include a spinal disc problem or a trigger point (see chapter 2 for more information) in the buttocks.

The symphysis pubis is the joint located at the front of the hip region in the groin area. It can become sprained by heavy or repetitive motion. Pain from this type of injury often occurs in the low back region, buttocks, or groin.

Injuries of the hip area are often the result of muscular imbalance in the body due to postural problems. It is critical to rebalance the muscles of the back and buttocks to prevent future injuries to the area. Exercise and postural activities are essential.

For Knee Injuries

Unfortunately, knee injuries are commonplace, both from trauma and overuse. An injury known as chondromalacia patella (or just chondromalacia for short) is the result of the cracking and breaking down of the smooth cartilage surface behind the kneecap. Pain is usually worse when there is pressure on the knee in a bent position. Treatment of this type of knee injury usually entails strengthening the muscles in the quadriceps (the front of the thigh) to rebalance the joint that is out of position.

There are two crescent-moon-shaped cartilages in the knee called menisci that act as shock absorbers for the body. Tears may result from twisting the knee while it is bent. Some injuries to the meniscus are treated by surgery, which entails removing the torn cartilage. These injuries may involve ligament damage as well. Treatment should involve rest, ice, and exercises to strengthen and balance the knee joints.

Ligament injuries in the knee should also be treated with the RICE procedure. Avoid activity too soon after knee injuries as it can worsen the problem. After a couple of weeks, begin gentle exercises to help strengthen the knees. Gradually, increase the level of exercise.

For Ankle Injuries

Most ankle injuries involve the ligaments on the outer side of the ankle. Use the RICE procedure immediately to help with pain, inflammation, and bruising. Wearing an ankle brace may give temporary support to the ankle. Treatment normally entails exercise on a "wobble board" that helps to strengthen the surrounding muscles.

Medical Approach to Joint Injuries

The typical medical approach to dealing with joint injuries is:

- non-steroidal anti-inflammatory medications (NSAIDs—see chapter 2 for more information);
- corticosteroids (see chapter 2);
- surgical repair; or
- replacement of damaged joints.

These treatments can have many harmful side effects. NSAIDs include aspirin, acetaminophen (Tylenol), ibuprofen (Advil), and others. Some of the possible side effects of these medications include: gastrointestinal bleeding and ulcers, gastrointestinal distress (heartburn, nausea, stomach pain, vomiting, diarrhea), headaches, dizziness and/or tinnitus. Over longer periods of time they can cause kidney and liver damage. NSAIDs have been shown to inhibit cartilage repair and even increase the rate of destruction of cartilage—the very problems many people take NSAIDs to help.

Corticosteroids deplete your body's immune system response, thereby making you more prone to infections of all kinds. In addition, they're harmful to the adrenal glands (the stress glands), and cause depression, high blood pressure, diabetes, cataracts, blurred vision, severe muscular weakness, ulcers, thinning of the skin, and osteoporosis.

As I mentioned in chapter 2, inflammation is a common symptom of many injuries. Any disorder that ends in "itis" means there is inflammation involved, for example, bursitis, arthritis, etc. Inflammation is the body's healthy response to infection, tissue damage or both. By sending increased amounts of white blood cells to the injured area, the body is better able to repair any damage. Without the inflammation process, injuries would not heal at all. Taking anti-inflammatory medications is therefore quite dangerous since it interferes with the natural healing process.

Arthritis and Bursitis

Arthritis is inflammation of the joints. There are two main types: osteoarthritis and rheumatoid arthritis. Osteoarthritis is the most common form and is also known as degenerative joint disease because of the loss of cartilage (the shock-absorbing gel-like material between joints). Rheumatoid arthritis is a chronic inflammatory condition that not only affects the joints, but the whole body.

Bursitis is inflammation of the bursa, a membrane that contains fluid and serves to lubricate the joints. It is usually less serious than arthritis, which is a chronic condition. Bursitis tends to be the acute result of overuse of a joint.

Injured joints are more prone to developing arthritis.

Foods That Affect Arthritis

You may be surprised to learn that some of the main aggravators of arthritis are foods. Some of the very substances we put into our body for nourishment actually worsen arthritis. I have already discussed some foods that alleviate or worsen inflammation in general. The following goes into detail about specific foods that aggravate or help the inflammation of the joints, namely arthritis and bursitis.

As early as 1766, an English medical text recommended cod liver oil to treat rheumatism and gout. By the mid-1800s it was regularly recommended for inflammation. While many people think it far-fetched that food could cause or lessen inflammation, they haven't been keeping up with the research that proves this phenomenon. In fact, leading specialists in arthritis often acknowledge that food may be the sole or leading cause of arthritic attacks.

In scientific studies, the main foods found to trigger or aggravate joint inflammation include:

- corn
- milk
- wheat
- meat
- Omega-6 vegetable oils (sunflower, safflower and canola)

On the other hand, according to scientific studies, the following are beneficial for arthritis symptoms:

- fatty fish
- ginger
- a vegetarian diet

Jean Carper, in her book, *Food: Your Miracle Medicine*, cites a study by British authority L. Gail Darlington. This study found that there are twenty foods that provoke or aggravate inflammation of the joints, particularly for people who are prone to arthritis.

With the worst culprits being at the top, the main foods that provoked symptoms are:

Aggravating Food	Percentage of Patients Affected
Corn	56
Wheat	54
Bacon/Pork	39
Oranges	39
Milk	37
Oats	37
Rye	34
Eggs	32
Beef	32
Coffee	32
Malt	27
Cheese	24
Grapefruit	24
Tomato	22
Peanuts	20
Sugar (from cane)	20
Butter	17
Lamb	17
Lemon	17
Soya	17

Natural Solutions for Inflamed Joints

Food is the best medicine for inflamed joints. There are many foods that are well-documented as anti-inflammatory. Some of the main ones include:

- fish rich in Omega-3, such as salmon, tuna and mackerel
- fatty acids, paricularly EPA (eicosapentaenoic acid)
- ginger
- turmeric
- cloves

Jean Carper, author of *Food: Your Miracle Medicine*, recounts the story of a woman who experienced total relief from severe rheumatoid arthritis upon beginning a vegetarian diet. In fact, she improved so significantly that she was able to eliminate her dependence on many drugs. Her physician, Dr. Fuhrman, initially put the woman on a fast and followed it with a vegetarian program. She now no longer requires the nine different medications she was taking to manage her symptoms and has regained physical strength and movement that was lost ten years earlier.

Many people suffering from arthritic symptoms can experience improvement by eliminating dairy products such as milk, butter, sour cream, yogurt, cottage cheese, cream, and cheese. To prove this fact, Dr. Richard Panush conducted a study on rabbits and was able to *produce* inflammatory synovitis in their joints by simply switching their water to milk. In an Israeli study, scientists observed more than a 50 percent reduction in the pain and swelling of arthritis when participants eliminated milk from their diet.

According to the research of Dr. Krishna C. Srivastava of Odense University in Denmark, ginger is superior to NSAIDs in alleviating pain and inflammation. NSAIDs work on one level—blocking the substances that cause inflammation. Ginger works on at least two mechanisms: 1) it blocks the formation of prostaglandins and leukotrienes; and 2) ginger has antioxidant properties that actually break down inflammation and acidity in the joints' synovial fluid.

Turmeric and cloves also fight inflammation effectively. Curcumin, the main therapeutic constituent of the spice turmeric, improved morning stiffness, walking time and joint swelling in 18 patients with rheumatoid arthritis. In fact, ingesting 1,200 mg of curcumin had the same therapeutic effect as 300 mg of the anti-inflammatory drug phenylbutazone.

When your joints heal from an injury it is imperative to be alert to any possible flare-ups of pain, since they can be linked to food sensitivities or allergies. Even with no underlying arthritis, certain foods can trigger joint pain in sensitive people.

I experienced this problem after I sustained car accident injuries. Suddenly, the joints affected would flare up on an almost ongoing basis. It appears to have been from consuming meat, too many Omega-6 fatty acids, and food sensitivities (which I wasn't even aware that I had). This was before I discovered the important dietary steps to take to make improvements.

I started a cleansing program that involved detoxifying my body. Inflammation and stress, among countless other things, create toxins in the body, many of which have an affinity for joints. The Eight-Week Injury-Healing Program results in cleansing the body while assisting it to repair injuries. When I reintroduced certain foods like dairy products, wheat, or had a misfortunate encounter with foods containing additives and colors, I would immediately experience increased pain and inflammation. Avoidance of these foods made a tremendous difference and greatly improved my recovery from joint injuries.

Keep in mind that most people have absolutely no idea that they might have food sensitivities. It is only AFTER ELIMINATING certain foods that they start to feel better over time. Some people notice immediate improvements while for others it takes a longer period of time.

I have had clients come to me who are surprised to learn that dairy products or food preservatives aggravate their joint pain. After attempting to remove dairy products they experienced no improvement. After examining their diets, I would frequently discover that these people were still eating cured meat (laden with preservatives), other meats (full of saturated fats that aggravate inflammation), baked goods with margarine or shortening, and salads in which the dressings are made from sunflower or safflower oil. So, making one small change is not enough if the rest of your diet is full of foods and chemicals that are known triggers of pain and inflammation. Sometimes ignorance is not bliss, nor is laziness or lack of effort going to improve one's health.

Dr. D.N. Golding, a rheumatologist at Princess Alexandra Hospital in Harlow, Essex, England, discovered something that he calls "allergic synovitis," which is inflammation of the synovial membrane that secretes fluid in the joint cavities to keep the joints lubricated and moving smoothly. Joint pain typically follows inflammation. The people most often struck with inflammation and pain are those with allergies, especially those who experience other allergic types of symptoms such as rashes, hives, and hay fever. Dr. Golding cites dairy products, including cheese and eggs as the most common culprits of "allergic synovitis."

As early as in 1943, a study showed that 20 percent of allergic patients had rheumatic pains as well.

Willow bark, which is the forerunner of aspirin, contains salicin and other salicylates, compounds that effectively diminish pain and inflammation. Use a tea brewed from up to one ounce (four tablespoons) of the dry, raw herb per day or as an ointment containing 240 mg of total salicin per day for as long as necessary.

Guggul gum (commiphora mukul) is an Ayurvedic herb used for arthritic diseases. You can take two to 10 capsules per day, 600 mg per capsule.

RICE Procedure for Injuries

The RICE procedure, consisting of rest, ice, compression and elevation is helpful for immediate attention to joint injuries, as I have already outlined in this chapter when describing specific injuries.

Aromatherapy for Joint Injuries

Connie and Alan Higley, authors of *Aromatherapy A-Z*, suggest that some of the best essential oils to lessen pain and improve healing of the joints include oils made from nutmeg, spruce, birch, or chamomile. Nutmeg, spruce and birch are best for aching joints or joint pain. Chamomile is suitable for joint inflammation. The oils should be diluted in a carrier oil such as almond, apricot kernel, grape seed, avocado, or hazelnut oil and applied directly on the injured area (provided there is no broken skin).

For a more complete list of essential oils, see Chapter 5.

Dealing with Dislocated Joints

The first course of action when dealing with a dislocation of a major joint is to seek medical attention. A dislocation may include injury to ligaments, tendons and nerves and should be immobilized. A dislocation to a major joint (shoulder, knee, elbow, jaw, ankle, etc.) is characterized by swelling, considerable pain and deformity to the injured area. Shock often accompanies this type of injury.

Arnica in mid- to high-range potencies can often assist with both the shock and immediate pain of the dislocation. Following relocation of the afflicted joint by an experienced medical practitioner, ruta can be administered in low- or mid-range potencies to deal with the trauma.

Bryonia (bryonia alba) is derived from the root of wild hops (also known as bryony or white bryony) and can be useful for swelling and pain resulting from slight movements of the relocated joint. It can be used in conjunction with arnica to address pain during the healing process.

Dealing with Sciatica

While this is a disorder affecting the nervous system, it is often the result of an injury or degeneration from an injury. The sciatic nerve is the main nerve in the leg and is connected to nerves in both the pelvis and the spine. Sciatica is frequently felt in the buttock region and thigh, usually on one side of the body. Sciatica occurs when there is unusual pressure on the nerve. This may be the result of degeneration from osteoarthritis, a prolapsed vertebral disk or, in some cases, ankylosing spondylitis, an unusual autoimmune disease. Sciatic pain often flares up when an individual bends, sneezes or coughs.

When sciatic pain is worse from sitting and it is difficult to straighten the leg, ammonium mur (ammonium chloratum) in low potencies such as 6c is recommended in half-hour doses for up to five hours. Common names for this mineral-derived remedy include sal ammoniac or ammonium chloride. Sciatica that is exacerbated by cold, damp weather resulting in numbness and weakness in the leg may be improved by colocynthis (cucumis colocynthis). Colocynthin is a substance found in a gourd known as bitter apple, bitter cucumber or colocynth. It causes severe cramps, and inflammation of the gastrointestinal tract if ingested. Samuel Hahnemann, the "father of homeopathy," found it effective for treating these symptoms, as well as neuralgia. It can be used in the same potencies and dosages suggested for ammonium mur. Rhus tox (rhus toxicodendron) is used when sciatica is relieved by heat and movement, stretching the limbs and rubbing the painful area. Rhus tox comes from the leaves of poison ivy or poison oak.

Dealing with Sprains

These injuries refer to damage to the ligaments. Ligaments are the fibrous, elastic connective tissues that surround joints. A sprain can refer to excessive stretching of the ligaments or, in the case of a severe sprain, the actual separation of the ligament from the joint.

Sprains are classified into three categories: first, second and third degree. First-degree sprains are the most common, resulting in tenderness and swelling around the injured joint. Second-degree sprains are identified with greater swelling and pain, as well as discoloration on the skin surrounding the joint. Joint movement may be limited with this injury. In addition to the symptoms above, a joint with a third degree sprain will be unstable. For example, a person may not be able to support their weight on a severely sprained ankle. While first- and second-degree sprains are commonly addressed through anti-inflammatory medication, rest, ice, compression, elevation and, later, heat, third-degree sprains should be evaluated and treated by a medical specialist.

In the case of homeopathic treatment of sprains, the homeopathic remedy may replace the anti-inflammatory medication. It can be used to combat pain, swelling and assist with the overall recovery. These remedies include arnica, bryonia or rhus tox, and ruta. As I have mentioned repeatedly, arnica is an excellent "first remedy" for most physical injuries, including sprains. A low to medium potency every 30 minutes for up to two hours, followed by three doses daily, will help combat the swelling and pain. If the injury is worsened by movement, bryonia is recommended in low to medium potencies in the same dosages as arnica. If the injured area feels better when it is moved, rhus tox is suggested in the same potencies and dosages as arnica. Ruta works best after the swelling and pain has subsided. It will promote healing of the ligaments and tendons and can be taken in 6x to 30x or 30c potencies every 30 minutes for up to four doses and three to four times daily until noticeable improvement takes place.

If an ankle is repeatedly sprained or easily sprained, ledum (ledum palustre) may be useful. This remedy is derived from wild rosemary (also known as marsh tea) and has been successfully used to address joints that are swollen, feel cold or make cracking noises when moved. Ledum may also be beneficial in cases of osteoarthritis.

Injury to joints and connective tissue was once believed to be irreparable. That is no longer the case. More recent research shows that the body can repair damage when the cells are properly nourished. Cartilage cells may multiply and create new, healthy collagen and cartilage, which are the major components of all connective tissue.

Assist your body in healing joint injuries by using the RICE procedure, eliminating damaging foods, adding healing foods and spices, exercising (when the injury has healed adequately), and using appropriate aromatherapy and homeopathic remedies.

4
EATING FOR HEALING

Healing Foods vs. Pharmaceutical Analgesics

When you consider the intense nature of pain and inflammation that can come from injuries, it may be hard to believe that the best remedies are the common foods found in your refrigerator. It may, in fact, be far more tempting to reach for a powerful prescription drug to eliminate the pain. I urge you to reconsider taking this action.

In the case of prescription pain medications, for example, they mask symptoms, that is what they are for. They prevent you from doing the right thing for yourself by giving you a sense of security. When the result, with pain medications, is no more pain, you assume there must be no more problem. Actually, the problem goes into hiding, which is why people continue to progress from one stage of the disease to the next.

In a 1996 issue of *Townsend Letter for Doctors* (*www.townsendletter.com*), the following was reported: "The biological action of every prescription drug can essentially be duplicated with nutritional supplements." The nutrients, however, do not share the extensive list of side effects that accompany most prescription and OTC drugs—particularly in the category of pharmaceutically prepared analgesics

Why Pain Is a Friend

Doctors write prescriptions for pain medications because people want fast and simple pain relief (or some other type of relief) without wanting to make changes to their lives, namely changing eating and lifestyle habits. But, the danger looms. Drug interactions and side effects, as well as contraindications, remain a serious problem in North America, which can frequently lead to death. Millions do not understand how to take their medications correctly, and abuse prescriptions, while doctors and pharmacists frequently do not communicate with one another, which can lead to misprescribing, duplicating prescriptions and healthcare error.

So, I urge you to stop EVERY time you want to pop a pain pill. Think of what your body is trying to tell you and LISTEN. "Pain," as Diamond clearly demonstrates, "is the body's most effective warning signal...Pain is your friend." How's that for a new concept? It may not feel comfortable. That is the whole idea. It may not be the friend you would like to have show up on your doorstep, but it is a friend nonetheless. Learning to view pain in a different way will serve you well for the rest of your life. Pain is the means by which the intelligence of the body brings a problem situation to your attention. Does pain get your attention? It should. Pain is also the body's attempt to heal itself. By masking the pain with OTC or prescription pain medications, you are simply avoiding the messages your body gives you.

Food as Medicine

You can overcome pain, inflammation, and injuries using totally natural means, the bulk of which should be the foods you choose to eat.

Foods are not simply for our enjoyment and nourishment, they are powerful healers in a vibrant multicolor disguise. Most people do not realize this fact because they are eating the wrong foods or not enough of the right foods. Before you think that I will have you on some starvation diet made up of only bland vegetables, keep reading. You are about to learn that the best healing remedies also taste fabulous (I cannot say that about any prescription medications). Plus, foods will not cause the nasty side effects common to pharmaceutical drugs.

Natural Anti-Inflammatories

Inflammation is the body's way of coping with an injury. It signals that the body is sending white blood cells to the area of the injury to fight infection, oxygenated blood to repair damage, and other fluids to cushion any damaged cells. This process is perfectly normal and healthy. However, when inflammation lasts for long periods of time or when low-grade inflammation occurs in the body, it is essential to get it under control using natural means. In fact, low-grade inflammation can result from oxidation within the blood vessel walls. Inflammation can even be a precursor to serious disease. That is one of the reasons why injured joints tend to be more vulnerable to disorders like arthritis. The damaged area incurs further damage through oxidation and inflammation.

Why Fats Are Deadly

The standard North American diet actually worsens inflammation because it is high in trans-fats or hydrogenated fats, sugar, refined flour, and food additives. Most packaged, processed, or prepared foods contain these incredibly harmful fats in the form of fried foods, shortening, lard, and even margarine, which many people believe is healthy. In actual fact, it is a toxic chemical that the body does not recognize as food. In addition to clogging arteries, it contributes to arthritic symptoms and worsens inflammation from injuries.

The typical diet, if it contains any essential fatty acids, usually includes fats from meat and poultry or healthier fats from nuts and seeds called Omega-6 fatty acids. While these fats are healthy in a ratio of 1:1 or even 2:1 of Omega 6s to Omega 3s (another essential fatty acid that the body must get from food), most people eat a 20:1 ratio. This excess worsens and even causes inflammation in the body. Omega-6 fatty acids are found in the highest concentrations in corn, sunflower, and safflower oils. Eating too many Omega-6 fatty acids in contrast to Omega-3 fatty acids will produce substances in the body that will trigger or worsen existing inflammation. This applies to everyone, not just people with sensitivities to these foods.

Consuming oils like corn oil, safflower oil, and sunflower oil or animals fed these fats in their diets can worsen inflammation in the body, aggravate arthritic pain, and negate the beneficial effects of fish and fish oils (more on this later). For example, if you eat a salad in which the dressing is made of one of these oils along with a piece of fatty fish, the oil in the salad will undo the benefits of eating the fish. Another example is tuna fish or sardines made into tuna salad or served on a sandwich alongside mayonnaise. The mayonnaise will counter any positive effects of eating the fish and lengthen or, worse, prevent the full healing of injuries in the body.

The oils with higher amounts of Omega-3 fatty acids include: flax oil (do not heat this oil—it is best reserved for salad dressings or as a topping for steamed vegetables or baked potatoes), canola oil, olive oil, and walnut oil. Other sources include dark greens like spinach and kale.

Sugar, white flour and food additives increase inflammation in the body. Decrease, or better yet, eliminate your contact with them. They are nutrition-less foods and chemicals that add no value to a diet. That does not mean you have to give up your favorite foods. As I will explain later, you can make healthy treats that actually PROMOTE healing instead of worsening the symptoms of injuries. I am including recipes in chapter 9 to help you get started on your Eight-Week Injury-Healing Program.

The Joy of Fish Oils

Two of the most common symptoms involved with injuries are pain and inflammation. There are many foods that are scientifically proven anti-inflammatories. The most popular are foods that contain Omega-3 fatty acids. Omega-3s are found in flax seeds and flax oil and fatty coldwater fish like salmon and tuna. Omega-3s convert in the body into hormone-like substances that decrease inflammation. These fatty acids are also found in canola and olive oil, raw walnuts, spinach, and kale.

According to Dr. Alfred D. Steinberg, an arthritis expert at the National Institute of Health, fish oil is an anti-inflammatory agent. Fish oil acts directly on the immune system by suppressing 40 to 55 percent of the release of cytokines, compounds known to destroy joints.

There are many studies that demonstrate that eating moderate amounts of fish or taking fish oil reduces inflammation, particularly for arthritis. Dr. Joel M. Kremer, M.D. conducted a double-blind study of 33 patients with multiple swollen and tender joints, fatigue and morning stiffness lasting for more than one half hour. When they took fish oil capsules for 14 weeks, their symptoms improved. Joint tenderness improved by more than one third and they were free of fatigue for over two and one half hours longer each day.

Dr. Kremer found that fish oils suppressed the body's production of leukotriene B4, the main inflammatory substance in the body and one that is considered largely responsible for arthritic symptoms. He observed that the lower the production of leukotriene B4, the fewer the number of tender joints.

Another study had similar results with fish oil and found that leukotrienes lessened within one month of supplementation with fish oil. When a person discontinues taking fish oil, leukotriene production increases again within one month.

Dr. Kremer suggests that the longer a person continues taking fish oil, the more rapid and intense improvements are. The daily amount used in the study was the equivalent of eating a seven-ounce serving of salmon or two cans of sardines per day.

The verdict: if you're fighting inflammation from your injury or if joint injuries have resulted in arthritis in your body, eat fish daily or supplement with fish or salmon oil capsules daily. It takes more fish oil to lessen arthritis than to prevent it. Since injured joints are prone to developing arthritis, consuming fish or fish oils is an excellent preventive and curative measure (if following a sensible diet like the one suggested here and a sensible lifestyle and exercise regime).

The Benefits of Berries

While many people opt for aspirin as their first course of action when they incur an injury, Muraleedharan Nair, Ph.D., professor of natural products and chemistry at Michigan State University, found that tart cherry extract is ten times more effective than aspirin at relieving inflammation. Only two tablespoons of the concentrated juice need to be taken daily for effective results. Later she found that sweet cherries, blackberries, raspberries, and strawberries have similar effects. Only two tablespoons of the concentrated juice need to be taken daily for effective results. Blueberries are excellent anti-inflammatory agents. They increase the amounts of compounds called heat-shock proteins that decrease as people age, thereby causing inflammation and damage, particularly in the brain. By eating blueberries regularly, research shows that these heat-shock proteins stop declining; inflammation lessens and pain decreases, not to mention that they just taste fabulous. When my mother quit smoking, she started eating frozen blueberries as her treat instead of cigarettes. Later, she told me about this newly found habit. Knowing about the research into the effectiveness of blueberries with inflammation and experiencing no shortage of the problem myself, I started eating frozen blueberries as a nightly dessert. Incidentally, I saw a rapid decline in pain and inflammation, plus my body started to feel lighter and movements freer. Frozen blueberries taste like blueberry sorbet. There are few treats as satisfying.

The Pluses of Fruits and Veggies

James Duke, Ph.D.; author of The Green Pharmacy, found more than 20 anti-inflammatory compounds in celery and celery seeds, including a substance called apigenin, which is powerful in its anti-inflammatory action. Incidentally, Hildegard von Bingen, writer, scientist, musician, nun and visionary, wrote about celery's anti-inflammatory properties over 900 years ago.

If you're not sure how to use celery seeds, add them to soups, stews or as a salt substitute in many recipes. One of my favorite foods as an appetizer instead of garlic bread is celery bread. Simply brush olive oil on whole grain bread (preferably not wheat) and sprinkle with celery seeds, bake in a 350-degree oven until golden-brown and serve as a tasty side dish.

Most colorful fruits and vegetables contain healing phytochemicals (plant chemicals) that reduce inflammation. Some of the notable ones include pineapple, which contains the powerful anti-inflammatory enzyme known as bromelain. Bromelain also helps with weight loss.

Specific food compounds known as flavonoids (also called Vitamin P) also help with healing and injuries. They increase the absorption of Vitamin C and have healing properties themselves. For example, flavonoids improve blood vessel health, which is important if blood vessels are involved in the injury you sustained. You will know if blood vessels are involved if you experience bruising or bleeding. Flavonoids have anti-inflammatory properties due to their antioxidant properties and their ability to act against histamines and other substances linked with inflammation, including prostaglandins and leukotrienes.

Tomatoes and bell peppers also contain about 20 anti-inflammatory substances each. I recommend eating tomatoes and peppers raw as much as possible because when they are cooked they become highly acidic. Pain, inflammation, and injuries worsen if the blood becomes acidic. This is yet another reason why a typical Western diet encourages disease and disorder. The typical Western diet is highly acidic, which in turn, acidifies the blood.

Diet helps regulate the body's inflammatory agents and avoiding certain types of food can elicit a powerful anti-inflammatory response in the body. What this means to you is that by eating a vegetarian or predominantly vegetarian diet (fish can be included in the diet if you prefer) high in critical nutrients found in spices like ginger, garlic, and onions; loaded with berries and cherries; and plenty of enzyme-rich raw fruits and vegetables, you will experience tremendous injury healing.

Foods to Avoid While Recovering from Injuries

The following foods aggravate pain and inflammation and therefore should not be consumed if your objective is healing:

- all processed, packaged, or fast foods;
- all hydrogenated fats (margarine, shortening, lard or products made with them such as cookies, pies, packaged foods, buns, etc.);
- all meat;
- all fried foods (French fries, onion rings, potato chips, nachos, hamburgers, etc.);
- all white sugar (and foods made from this sweet);
- other sugars (brown sugar, cane sugar, turbinado sugar, demarrara sugar, molasses, beet sugar, date sugar—although a small amount of honey is permitted as is stevia, an herb that is naturally one thousand times sweeter than sugar);
- all synthetic sweeteners (Nutrasweet, saccharin, aspartame, etc.);
- salt (use Celtic sea salt instead and limit sodium intake and note: Celtic sea salt is not the same as sea salt);
- all food additives (colors, flavor enhancers, stabilizers, preservatives, etc.);
- all dairy products (yogurt, ice cream, cottage cheese, butter, cheese, etc.);
- all wheat products (wheat, even whole wheat is very acidifying and can counter the benefits of the program);
- coffee and black tea (green tea and herbal teas are permitted);
- all soft drinks, sweetened juices, fruit punch and other sweetened beverages; and
- all alcohol.

Foods to Eat While Recovering from Injuries

The following foods are beneficial to assist with healing injuries:

- raw fruits and vegetables;
- fatty fish (like salmon, mackerel, herring, sardines, and tuna);
- flax oil, walnut oil, hemp oil, or extra virgin olive oil;
- spices like turmeric, garlic, cloves, onions, ginger, celery seeds, turmeric, chili peppers, licorice (the herb), peppermint, and paprika;
- celery and lots of raw and cooked vegetables;
- fresh, raw vegetable and fruit juices (made at home in a juicer);
- plenty of raw tomatoes and bell peppers;

- plenty of raw apples, pineapple, berries like blueberries, blackberries, raspberries, strawberries, and cherries;
- fresh raw nuts, especially walnuts and almonds (including raw almond milk);
- leafy greens like spinach, dandelion greens and kale;
- whole grains and legumes; and
- soy foods (soy milk, tofu, but not the heavily processed soy derivatives like hot dogs, luncheon meats, etc.).

The Case for (Almost-Total) Vegetarianism

If you're suffering from any type of inflammation from your injuries, there are three great reasons to give up meat, says Jean Carper, author of *Food: Your Miracle Medicine*.

1. Meat contains the type of fat that stimulates production of inflammatory agents in the body.

2. Meat may produce "allergic" reactions that incite arthritis flare-ups because of individual reactions, probably inherited.

3. Some meats, particularly cured meats, such as bacon, ham, hot dogs and cold cuts, contain preservatives and other chemicals that trigger allergic arthritic reactions in some individuals. This is in addition to the inflammatory properties of the meat's fat. I was tempted to add a fourth reason: no one ever died of mad broccoli disease. Avoid meat while healing since saturated fats, particularly those found in bacon, pork and beef, stimulate the inflammatory process.

A study by Norwegian researchers in 1991 found that meatless diets relieved arthritic symptoms in nine out of ten patients. That is a 90 percent effectiveness rate. There is no medical treatment that can even come close to having such a high effectiveness rate.

Carper recounts another study that demonstrates the benefits of a vegetarian diet for people suffering from joint damage: "Jens Kjeldsen-Kragh, M.D., of the Institute of Immunology and Rheumatology at the National Rheumatism Hospital of Oslo, found that switching to a vegetarian diet resulted in better grip strength and much less pain, joint swelling and tenderness and morning stiffness in about 90 percent of a group of arthritic subjects, compared with the control group eating an ordinary diet. The subjects noticed improvement within a month, and it lasted throughout the entire year-long study."

At the beginning of the program, participants ate a detoxifying type of diet for one week. It consisted of herbal teas, vegetable broths, and carrot, beet, celery and potato juices. For the next three to five months, they ate a vegan diet (no animal products at all, which means no meat, fish, milk, poultry, and eggs). They also avoided gluten (found in many grains, particularly wheat), refined sugar, citrus fruits, strong spices and preservatives. Next they added foods back one by one. If they observed a "flare-up" within a 24 to 48-hour period after eating the food, they rejected that food for one week and then reintroduced it again. If after the second attempt to include it in their diet they saw another flare-up of symptoms, they avoided the food for the remainder of the study.

Dr. Kjeldsen-Kragh concluded that approximately 70 percent of people saw improvement in inflammation and pain because they avoided the wrong kinds of fats, namely from meat, which is well known to worsen the inflammation process. Others saw improvements because they excluded foods to which they were sensitive or allergic.

Ginger has been used for thousands of years as part of Ayurvedic medicine in India as a natural anti-inflammatory food. Dr. Krishna C. Srivastava of Odense University in Denmark, a world-renowned researcher on the therapeutic effects of spices, discovered how ginger works. Dr. Srivastava tested small amounts of ginger daily for three months on a group of arthritic patients. The majority of people in the study experienced less pain, swelling, and morning stiffness from eating higher amounts of ginger.

Jean Carper's book, *Food: Your Miracle Medicine* includes a story by Dr. Srivastava of a 50-year-old Asian auto mechanic who ingested ginger daily within one month of a diagnosis of arthritis. Every day he lightly cooked 50 grams (1 and 3/4 ounces) of fresh ginger with his foods. After three months of regular ginger consumption, he was completely free of pain, inflammation and swelling and remained so for ten years.

Dr. Srivastava successfully treated 50 patients with ginger over a two-year period as well. He recommends five grams of fresh ginger (1/6 of an ounce) or 1/3 of a teaspoonful of dried ginger taken three times per day. He suggests that ginger is more effective than NSAIDs (see chapter 2 for additional information).

NSAIDs work on one level, blocking the substances that cause inflammation. Ginger works on at least two mechanisms: 1) It blocks the formation of prostaglandins and leukotrienes; and 2) Ginger has antioxidant properties that actually break down inflammation and acidity in the joints' synovial fluid.

Turmeric and cloves also fight inflammation effectively. Curcumin, the main therapeutic constituent of the spice turmeric, improved morning stiffness, walking time and joint swelling in 18 patients with rheumatoid arthritis. In fact, ingesting 1,200 mg of curcumin had the same therapeutic effect as 300 mg of the anti-inflammatory drug phenylbutazone.

An Indian study found that regular garlic-eaters often got relief from joint pain, particularly those people with osteoarthritis. During the study, the people who obtained relief ate two to three cloves of raw or cooked garlic daily. Garlic affects prostaglandin levels in the body, thereby lessening inflammation.

Capsaicin, the ingredient that makes hot peppers hot, has long been used in ointments and creams to ease the pain of arthritis. Now research shows that this ingredient is a local anesthetic (when applied directly to an affected area) and a powerful painkiller. It works on two premises: 1) It drains nerve cells of something called substance P which relays pain sensations to the central nervous system; and 2) It blocks the perception of pain.

Pain is your body's way of letting you know that something is wrong. It does not only occur in localized areas; rather, it travels by way of the spinal cord and nervous system, thereby sending pain messages to the brain. Many sensations travel the same pathway as pain. In fact, like a highway system, numerous sensations travel the same road. The speed of the sensation determines how quickly the message gets to the brain. Pain actually travels this pathway quite slowly. Dull pain travels approximately one-half mile to two miles per second. Sharp or burning pain travels at approximately five to 30 miles per second. Non-painful touch such as acupressure or massage travels at 35 to 75 miles per second.

Much like a sprint race where the fastest runner crosses the line first, the fastest sensation identified by the body displaces pain. This is one of the reasons why using a substance that creates a burning sensation works. It "outruns" most types of pain in the speed with which it registers to the brain.

If there is one critical factor to consider when healing from injuries, it is consistency. A person must eat or supplement his or her diet with the substances that aid in healing and reducing inflammation on a REGULAR basis. The same is true with the foods to avoid. These foods must be avoided on a REGULAR basis. As a person heals, his or her diet may not need to be quite as strict but in the short term a person should stick with the *Healing Injuries the Natural Way* program for the best results.

The Healing Power of Enzymes in Raw Foods

The most powerful approach to healing injuries is through nutrition. I am not referring to the Four Food Groups or the Food Pyramid. I am talking about foods that heal. Many people eat solely because food tastes good. I am not suggesting that you give up food you enjoy; rather, learn to prepare food that has healing properties in a way that it tastes fabulous.

This may seem contradictory but it is not. The most healing food you can find is in raw fruits and vegetables for two reasons:

1. Raw fruits and vegetables (along with raw, unsalted nuts and seeds) contain powerful substances called enzymes. Enzymes are the basis of all life. If you destroyed all enzymes on the planet, all life would disappear as well. Enzymes are essential for healing injuries.

2. Many other nutrients like vitamins are destroyed in the cooking process, making raw foods the healthiest choice for healing because of their higher nutrient content.

I am not suggesting that you have to become a raw foods vegetarian to heal from your injury unless you want to. I am merely saying that by eating at least 50 percent of every meal in a natural, raw state, you enable your body to heal faster, more completely, and you will feel great.

Eating a high raw diet is actually simple. Eat a couple pieces of fruit in the morning for breakfast before eating toast, cereal, or another breakfast food. At lunch, eat a large, raw salad with a dressing made of cold-pressed oils (full of Omega-3 fatty acids; more on this topic to follow) along with your soup or sandwich or other lunchtime food. At dinner, eat another raw salad along with your dinner foods. If you want snacks between meals or before bed, eat some raw fruit or drink some freshly pressed veggie juices or fruit smoothies. In this simple way you will get your raw food content up to 50 percent of your overall diet or more.

Mother Nature's Power Healing Foods

Salads do not have to consist of iceberg lettuce and a couple slices of starchy tomato topped with totally unhealthy ranch dressing. Actually, eating this way will only prolong your healing time and worsen any pain or inflammation you may be dealing with. There are few nutrients in this type of salad. As well, the store-bought dressing is usually full of trans-fats (dangerous substances that occur when oils are heated excessively) that CAUSE inflammation.

Salads can be gourmet meals in themselves. I suggest making your salad the focal point of your meal. You can do this by being creative in your approach to them. I compiled the following list of ingredients to consider for salads and to prevent boredom from eating them regularly:

- mixed greens (mesclun)
- romaine lettuce
- Boston lettuce
- leaf lettuce
- radicchio
- pea shoots
- alfalfa sprouts
- broccoli sprouts
- onion sprouts
- clover sprouts
- mung bean sprouts
- chick peas
- kidney beans
- pinto beans
- lima beans
- Great Northern beans
- any other type of legume
- sliced strawberries
- apple slices
- orange slices
- grapefruit slices
- avocado;
- green peppers
- red peppers
- yellow peppers
- finely chopped broccoli
- cucumber
- olives
- edible flowers
- grated carrots
- fresh peas
- grated cabbage
- chopped parsley
- chopped cilantro (coriander)
- mushrooms (raw or cooked)

- green onion
- raspberries
- blueberries
- celery

   Dressings can be made from cold-pressed oils such as extra-virgin olive oil, walnut oil, flax oil, coconut oil, or a blend of oils known as Udo's Blend (available in most health food stores). You can add freshly squeezed lemon or lime juice (bottled concentrate does not count), apple cider vinegar (make sure it has a live culture in it which means there will be some sediment in the bottom of the bottle), balsamic vinegar, red or white wine vinegar (in moderation). I have included some salad dressing recipes later in the book to help you get started.

The Healing Food Pyramid

Now that you've learned some of the essential foods to incorporate into your diet if you're trying to heal from either an acute or chronic injury, let's put it all together. I developed the Healing Food Pyramid as part of my quest for healing my injuries and my many years of research into foods that heal.

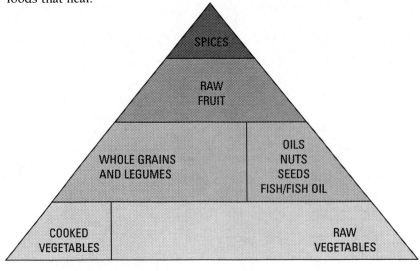

As you can see from the Healing Food Pyramid diagram, the bulk of your foods should be eaten in a raw state. There are countless ways to prepare raw fruits and vegetables and a multitude of ingredients that you can easily incorporate into salads. You will find some wonderful healing recipes in chapter 9. Most of the raw foods you eat should be vegetables and freshly pressed vegetable juices. A lesser amount of raw foods can include cold-pressed flax, olive, hemp, or walnut oil. Nuts and seeds should be eaten raw and unsalted.

To help you with your food choices, please use the Healing Foods Chart that follows which lists the best foods for each category of the Healing Food Pyramid and the top anti-inflammatory and anti-pain foods.

Healing Foods Chart*

Top Anti-Inflammatory and Anti-Pain Spices	Raw Fruit	Whole Grains** & Legumes	Oils***, Nuts****, Seeds, Fish & Fish Oils	Vegetables (Mostly Raw)	Top Anti-Inflammatory & Anti-Pain Foods	Foods with Natural Aspirin to Counter Pain	Top Calcium-Rich Body-Alkalizing Foods (in order of calcium potency)
Turmeric	Pineapple	Millet	Walnut oil	Mesclun	Cherries	Blueberries	Sesame
Celery	Papaya	Quinoa	Flax oil	(mixed	and cherry	Cherries	seeds
seeds	Mango	Brown	Hemp oil	greens)	juice	Dried	Seaweed,
Garlic	Lemon	rice	X-virgin	Romaine	Blueberries	currants	agar
Ginger	Lime	Spelt	olive oil	lettuce	Celery	Curry	Seaweed,
Cloves	Grapefruit	Kamut	Walnuts	Boston	Tomatoes	powder	dulse
Chili	Orange	Kidney	Hazelnuts	lettuce	(raw)	Dates	Collard
peppers	Kiwi	beans	Almonds	Radicchio	Bell pepper	Gherkins	leaves
(capsaicin)	Grapes	Garbanzo	Pecans	Pea shoots	(raw)	Licorice	Kale leaves
Licorice	Rhubarb	beans	Pistachios	Alfalfa	Pineapple	herb	Turnip
(herb)	Pears	Lentils	Sunflower	sprouts	Fatty fish	Paprika	greens
Peppermint	Apples	Lima beans	seeds	Broccoli	(salmon,	Prunes	Almonds**
Paprika	Avocado	Pinto beans	Pumpkin	sprouts	tuna,	Rasp-	***
Onion	Blueberries	Romano	seeds	Onion	mackerel	berries	Soy beans
	Cherries	beans	Sesame	sprouts	& herring)		Hazelnuts
	Black-		seeds	Clover	Flax oil		(filberts)
	berries		Salmon	sprouts	Walnuts		Brazil
	Rasp-		Mackerel	Mung bean	and walnut		nuts*****
	berries		Herring	sprouts	oil		Parsley
	Straw-		Tuna	Avocado	Spinach		Collard
	berries			Green/red/	Kale		stems
				yellow	Dandelion		Dandelion
				peppers	Apples		greens
				Broccoli	Onion		Mustard
				Cucumber	Dried		greens
				Carrots	currants		Kale stems
				Peas	Dates		Watercress
				Cabbage	Gherkins		Pepper
				Sweet	(small		(red hot)
				potatoes	cucum		Chick peas
				Yams	bers)		Sunflower
				Fennel	Prunes		seeds
				Bok choy	(unsul		Beet
				Fiddle-	phured)		greens
				heads	Rasp-		Mung bean
				Tomatoes	berries		sprouts
				(raw)	Black-		Brocolli
				Celery	berries		Fennel

Please note the following in reference to the preceding chart:

*   Do not assume that if a particular fruit or vegetable or berry does not appear on this list that it shouldn't be eaten or has no healing properties. I simply tried to include all the top ones in each category.

**   Avoid wheat products since they're very acidic and many people are sensitive to them. If you're celiac or have gluten sensitivity, you can still eat healthily following the remainder of the Healing Food Pyramid.

***   All oils should be cold-pressed and ideally bought in a health food store.

****   Avoid peanuts since they tend to contain many aflatoxins (mold-like substances), which aggravate joints and inflame tissues.

***** Nuts are only alkalizing if they are raw and unsalted.

5

NUTRITIONAL SUPPLEMENTS AND NATURAL REMEDIES

$\int$upplementing with specific nutrients and herbs can improve healing and lessen pain and inflammation. There are many high-quality supplements that are proven in study upon study to be effective in healing pain, inflammation, or injury. I have compiled information about some of the most effective proven ones. There may be many others that are not found within these pages.

Natural Remedies to Combat Pain and Inflammation

Sometimes proven remedies do not work outside of the studies. Typically this happens for two reasons. The first is that most people buy the cheapest, synthetic brand they can find in their local pharmacy or health food store. Oh sure, the label says "all natural" so they're duped into believing this product will help them. Many of these supplements are synthetic chemicals supplied by none other than the major pharmaceutical drug manufacturers. Because they're synthetic, the body rarely even recognizes them and does not utilize them. Typically they're also full of fillers. Many supplements do not even contain the ingredients listed on the label.

The second reason is that people take them on and off for a week or two and then claim "they do not work." Well, high-quality supplements typically need to be taken regularly (read daily, sometimes two or three times per day) for a minimum of several months. Also, deciding whether or not they work based on symptom relief is the wrong "paradigm" for supplements. Most people can't *feel* what's going on in their more than 120 trillion cells; nutritional supplements rarely work directly on symptoms.

Yet the sole purpose of OTC and prescription pain medication is to mask symptoms. Nutritional supplements go to work on the problem areas to attempt healing. Symptoms usually improve over time.

A 55-year-old adult cannot expect two weeks of supplementation with a single herb to alleviate years of bodily abuse and toxic build-up. Even if an injury was only sustained recently, the body may have been suffering tremendous insult through the accumulation of toxins. These toxins are then drawn to the "weakest link" in the body—the injured area—thereby lessening the effectiveness of healing. This is particularly true if a person pops an herbal pill daily while still eating steak and French fries, slapping margarine on toast, and occasionally eating a limp tomato on an iceberg lettuce salad or a heap of boiled carrots slathered in butter. Our typical diet in North America has few redeeming qualities and many more inflammatory effects.

The Importance of Essential Fatty Acids (EFAs)

Essential fatty acids are critical to balancing inflammation and pain in the body since they're the precursors of chemical messengers called prostaglandins.

Prostaglandins regulate inflammation. They're made from Omega-3 and Omega-6 fatty acids. Both are required. Most people are quite deficient in Omega-3 fatty acids. This can cause inflammation to go unchecked in the body. As you discovered in Chapter 4, Omega-3 fatty acids are found in the oils of cold-water fish, such as salmon, mackerel, and herring, as well as nuts and seeds like flax, hemp, walnut. While a person should strive to get as many Omega-3 fatty acids in the diet as possible, sometimes if there is severe inflammation the requirements may be too high to make this possible. In that case, supplementation may be helpful as well. I highly recommend that you try to make sources of EFAs a regular part of your diet. For those people who do not like the taste, they are easy to sneak into a fruit smoothie made with frozen banana (instead of dairy products for creaminess). You can also supplement with high-quality salmon oil, EFA blends, or cod liver oil capsules.

The Benefits of Glucosamine Sulphate

Derived from the shells of shellfish, glucosamine sulphate has been proven in tests to alleviate the pain of joint inflammation when taken consistently for a minimum of two weeks and sometimes longer. In clinical trials, glucosamine sulphate has proven more effective than any non-steroidal anti-inflammatory drug (NSAID). No drug can match its ability to halt the deterioration of joints. In one study of arthritic knees glucosamine sulphate, taken in dosages of 1,500 mg per day over three years, prevented further deterioration of the knees. Not a drug on this planet can do that. This was the effect on ALL the participants in the study. Glucosamine sulphate works when taken consistently over long periods of time.

Vitamin C with Bioflavonoids

When you peel into an orange, lemon, lime or grapefruit, you will not only get a taste explosion, you will get a powerful dose of Vitamin C along with partnering nutrients called bioflavonoids. The bulk of bioflavonoids are found in the white pith surrounding the orange, so be sure to leave some of it on (even if the taste is slightly bitter). Since Vitamin C is found in nature alongside bioflavonoids, if you're going to supplement your diet, it is best to take Vitamin C that contains bioflavonoids as well. This helps the body recognize it to utilize it better. Taking these nutrients speeds healing when taken at therapeutic levels, which can vary from 500 mg to several grams daily. If you opt for several grams daily, spread the dose out throughout the day or risk experiencing mild diarrhea.

Essential Nutrients for Healing Bones

As mentioned in chapter 1, there are many critical nutrients for bone health. They can be obtained through eating a well-rounded diet like the one suggested as part of the Eight-Week Injury-Healing Program. However, should you wish to supplement with them, the main bone strengthening nutrients include: boron, calcium, manganese, magnesium, phosphorus, potassium, silica, zinc, Vitamin A, Vitamins B—folic acid (B9), Vitamin B-6, and Vitamin B-12, Vitamin C, Vitamin D3 (cholecalciferol), Vitamin K, betaine hydrochloric acid, glucosamine sulphate, and ipiflavone (7-isopropoxy-isoflavone).

Herbal Therapy

There are many herbs that have been proven to lessen inflammation. Some of these include: willow bark, meadowsweet, feverfew, ginger, bupleurum, cat's claw, chinese skullcap, yucca, and devil's claw. Adding one or more of these herbs to your health regime will yield better results.

Herbs like these that reduce inflammation also tend to be effective at lessening pain. Have patience with them, unlike OTC and prescription pain medications that work quickly to stop chemical processes (usually accompanied by serious side effects), herbs sometimes take a little time. It may even require one to two weeks to notice improvements. Keep in mind that OTC and prescription pain medications stop symptoms but don't heal the body. Herbs usually work on healing the source of the problem, thereby lessening or stopping symptoms. Going straight to the root of the problem and helping it to heal is far more effective in the long term. Sometimes, the herbs actually improve mobility of the joints and muscles along with lessening pain and inflammation.

If you're currently taking any medication, have any health concerns or are pregnant, consult your physician or an herbalist before taking any herbal medicine.

Willow Bark and Meadowsweet

Willow bark and meadowsweet are two herbs that contain salicylic acid (the active ingredient in aspirin). However, the plants have far fewer, if any, side effects. Aspirin, on the other hand, is a well-known stomach irritant. Herbalists recommend taking willow bark or meadowsweet for many of the same symptoms for which you might consider taking aspirin (not while taking aspirin, however). Take two cups of willow bark or meadowsweet tea or one to two droppersfull of the tincture of the plants per day to lessen pain and inflammation. If you have stomach problems, use meadowsweet since herbalists even recommend using it to treat the pain of ulcers.

The plants appear to decrease the levels of prostaglandins, which are hormones that are manufactured in the body. For some reason, the body may manufacture too many of these hormones, resulting in increased pain. High levels of prostaglandins are typically implicated in most injuries, arthritis, migraines, and menstrual cramps.

Both willow bark and meadowsweet can be found in capsules or tablets at health food stores or from your local herbalist.

Feverfew

Feverfew reduces pain and inflammation by decreasing prostaglandins, according to numerous studies. Often, feverfew is more effective than aspirin. It contains different compounds than willow bark and meadowsweet, yet according to several American studies it also stops inflammation and its resulting pain by reducing prostaglandin levels in the body. If you do not get relief from willow bark or meadowsweet, try fever-few and vice versa. Experimenting with the herbs is the best way to deter-mine which one(s) will be most effective for your injury symptoms. Keep in mind though that it may take some time to notice symptom reduction.

If you suffer from migraines you may find feverfew helpful in migraine prevention. It may take ingesting two tablets of standardized feverfew extract daily for thirty days before you will notice improvement.

Ginger

Ginger also reduces prostaglandin levels in the body and has been wide-ly used in India to treat pain and inflammation. A study by Indian researchers found that when people who were suffering from muscular pain were given ginger, they all experienced some improvement. No one experienced any negative side effects, including people who supplement-ed their diets with ginger for more than two years.

The recommended dosage of ginger is between 500 and 1,000 mgs per day. Higher doses bring faster and better relief. In addition to reliev-ing pain, supplementation with ginger brings increased blood flow to the injured and inflamed area, thereby improving healing. Gingerroot increases circulation to muscles and is beneficial for soft tissue injuries or damage. Take between one to ten grams per day.

Bupleurum

Bupleurum (bupleurum falcatum) is a Chinese herb that has a long rep-utation for its effectiveness at reducing or relieving inflammation. It stim-ulates the pituitary and adrenal glands to increase natural production of hormones (like cortisone) that reduce inflammation and pain caused by injuries or arthritic conditions. Ginseng and licorice root work well in combination with bupleurum since they have similar effects but also enhance the functioning of the immune system.

Cat's Claw

This South American herb is known primarily for its immune system enhancing qualities, but has more recently been found to reduce inflam-mation. It grows claw-like stems that give the plant its odd name. Peruvian natives have used this herb for centuries. It is an excellent rem-edy for inflammatory disorders like arthritis and injuries where anti-inflammatory herbs are required.

Chinese Skullcap

Used extensively in China and Russia, Chinese skullcap has been recently found to be a more effective anti-inflammatory than ibuprofen and aspirin. In addition, it helps increase blood flow to the inflamed area, thereby increasing the speed of healing.

Yucca

Also an excellent herb for inflammation, yucca was found to be remarkably effective for arthritis in a French study. Participants took 1 and 1/2 grams of yucca per day and about 90 percent of them reported that the intensity of their pain decreased during the duration of the study.

Devil's Claw

This plant garners its name from its large fruit that grow in the shape of a large claw-like hand. Devil's claw has a long history of efficacy when used for arthritis, back pain, and inflammatory disorders. It can be taken as an herbal tea, in capsules or tablets, or as an ointment to rub on the painful areas.

Turmeric

Turmeric (curcuma has longa) is the yellow spice commonly used in Indian food. In research it has been shown to be a more effective anti-inflammatory than steroid medications when dealing with acute inflammation. Its main therapeutic ingredient is curcumin, which has been shown to deplete nerve endings of substance P, a pain neurostransmitter. Research shows that curcumin suppresses pain through a similar mechanism as drugs like COX-1 and COX-2 inhibitors (without the harmful side effects).

For acute episodes, people can take up to four tablespoons of turmeric mixed into water or honey per day. I find the honey-turmeric mixture to be far more palatable than taking turmeric in water or juice. For ongoing concerns, one teaspoon per day is sufficient to lessen pain. Turmeric can also be ingested in capsule form. In that case, choose a standardized extract with 1,500 mg of curcumin content per day. There are no known undesirable effects, even with large doses.

Curcumin is effective for bone, soft tissue and joint pain and inflammation.

Cayenne Pepper

Cayenne improves circulation and reduces pain. Take up to three 500 mg capsules per day. Be aware that some people find even a single capsule causes a burning sensation in the stomach. You can also use cayenne sprinkled on food with 1/4 teaspoon being the equivalent of approximately 400 mg.

Kava

Kava (piper methysticum) is an analgesic whose potency ranks between aspirin and morphine. It is a muscle relaxant and sleep aid but it does not create the negative morning symptoms linked to tranquillizers. Take kava in an alcohol-based tincture (85 percent alcohol), one teaspoon at bedtime and working up to one tablespoon. Because kava has been linked to liver damage, use it only under the guidance of a healthcare practitioner.

Ginkgo Biloba

In a 2002 study using ginkgo biloba and coenzyme Q-10, 64 percent of participants taking 200 mg of CoQ-10 and 200 mg of ginkgo extract daily for 84 days found improvement from fibromyalgia symptoms. Ginkgo is also effective for other soft tissue damage.

Boswellia Gum (Indian Frankincense)

Frankincense or boswellia gum has anti-inflammatory and pain relieving properties and may even help protect cartilage against injury. It is especially helpful in dealing with bursitis and arthritis. Use a standardized 65 percent boswellic acid product, 300 to 1,200 mg per day.

Guggul Gum

Guggul gum (commiphora mukul) is an Ayurvedic herb used for arthritic diseases. You can take two to ten capsules per day, 600 mg per capsule.

Aromatherapy for Healing Injuries

There are many essential oils that are effective for healing injuries, so I had to limit my list to the following seven well-established and easy-to-find ones. Do not use essential oils on broken skin and consult an aromatherapist if you're uncertain about any of the suggested remedies.

- Black pepper oil: in small amounts topically for healing joint, nerve or muscular pain.

- Ginger oil: as an essential oil applied topically to the skin, ginger stimulates circulation and is helpful for muscular pains and stiffness.
- Lavender oil: both a pain reliever and relaxant, lavender is good for sprains, muscle aches and stiffness.
- Lemongrass oil: useful for muscle aches and pains.
- Marjoram oil: can be used for bruises, sprains, muscle aches and stiffness.
- Rosemary oil: has anti-pain properties, is a relaxant and is useful for muscular and nerve pain.
- White camphor oil: use only white camphor (not brown or yellow since these are toxic) in the treatment of sprains, muscular pain, and stiffness.

Homeopathy for Healing Injuries

Homeopathic remedies have been used to treat illness and injury for over two centuries. The word "homeopathy" is derived from the Greek *homois*, which can be translated as "similar" and *pathos*, which can be translated as "suffering." Simply put, homeopathic remedies are chosen for their ability to create symptoms in a person's body—symptoms similar to those the person is experiencing as a result of an illness or injury.

The homeopathic theory is based on two premises: "like cures like" and "less is more." The former refers to the Law of Similars that states that the substances that provoke specific symptoms in a person's body can also demonstrate curative properties on similar symptoms. The "less is more" theory relates to Hahnemann's discovery that, the more one dilutes a remedy, the longer and more effectively it appears to work on the afflicted person. Some homeopathic remedies are so significantly diluted, that it becomes questionable whether a single molecule of the substance from which it was derived remains. Yet this is the secret to the remedies' potency. Hahnemann developed specific guidelines for a process he termed "potentization," to ensure the full strength of the substance could be released into the remedy and, of course, into the person using the remedy.

Homeopathy works best not only when the correct remedy is chosen for the condition, but when the correct potency is chosen as well. The scale of dilution determines this. Remedies are prepared according to one of two scales. In the decimal (x) scale, the dilution is 1:10. In the centesimal (c) scale the dilution factor is 1:100. For example, a remedy with

12x after the name has been diluted 12 times on the decimal scale. A remedy with 30c after the name has been diluted 30 times on the centesimal scale. Remedies may also be diluted on the millesimal (m) and quinquagintamillesimal (lm) scales, which are 1:1000 and 1:50,000 respectively. Homeopathic practitioners in very specific cases, such as potent single-dose treatment and chronic cases, use these extremely high dilutions. They should not be taken by individuals without first consulting a skilled practitioner.

Modern scientific research on the efficacy of homeopathic remedies has simply proven what many health practitioners have known for many years— homeopathy offers for many ailments a safe, non-toxic alternative to both over-the-counter and prescription drugs. In fact, prior to the prolific spread of drugs like penicillin, homeopathic treatment was widely used in North America and it has enjoyed a remarkable renaissance over the last decade. The United States Food and Drug Administration (USFDA) recognizes the legal status of homeopathy as approved drugs, based on those listed in the *Homeopathic Pharmacopoeia of the United States*. In Europe, homeopathy has maintained its popularity since its modern discovery by Samuel Christian Hahnemann (1755-1843), a German physician and chemist. And India is home to more homeopathic medical colleges and hospitals than any other nation, according to Lyle W. Morgan, author of *Homeopathic Treatment of Sports Injuries*.

In addition to its reported healing properties, homeopathy's strength is its accessibility. Most homeopathic remedies do not require a prescription and can be purchased directly at a pharmacy or a health food store. However, it is recommended that an individual consult with a health practitioner experienced in homeopathic treatment and remedies prior to using them.

Homeopathy can be used for virtually any health problem. Homeopathics are available as both formulas and single remedies. Formulas are often marketed for specific problems, such as colds or allergies. They are usually combinations of remedies in lower potencies. Single remedies are usually based on symptoms rather than "named" illnesses or disorders. As a result, a single remedy can be very powerful when the correct one is identified and delivered in an appropriate potency, which may be higher than those found in a formula.

Homeopathic remedies are usually in pill form, which are held under the tongue until they dissolve. They can also come in the form of tinctures that are also held under the tongue before swallowing. Certain homeopathic remedies are available for topical application in the form of ointments, gels and sprays. Ointments in a petroleum base will reduce the skin's ability to breathe and rid itself of toxins and are not recommended.

The following is a list of potential homeopathic remedies for common injuries.

Homeopathic Treatment for Bone Bruises

Ruta (ruta graveolens) is an effective remedy for bone bruises and connective tissue damage, such as injuries to ligaments and joints. Repetitive strain injuries may also be improved with ruta. Common names for the plant from which ruta is derived are "rue" or "herb of grace," a spindly, yellow-flowering herb native to dry, sunny regions in the Mediterranean.

If ruta does not improve the symptoms within the first 24 hours, symphytum (symphytum officinale) may be used. This remedy promotes bone healing and is derived from comfrey, a plant also known as knitbone. Both ruta and symphytum can be obtained in pill and ointment form. While all potencies are effective, the lower potencies can typically be taken for a longer period of time.

Homeopathic Treatments for Soft Tissue Bruises

A bruise or contusion is a soft tissue injury. The discoloration of the skin surface is linked to the rupture of small blood vessels in the tissues beneath the skin surface. This rupture has caused blood and other fluids to leak into the tissues. Arnica (arnica montana) is an effective remedy for contusions. In fact, arnica is the primary remedy for virtually all cases of physical injury due to its ability to relieve pain, reduce inflammation and assist with shock. The plant's healing properties, unlike its many names (leopard's bane, mountain daisy, sneezewort, and mountain tobacco) have been recognized for centuries. Arnica can be taken in doses of 30x or 30c every hour until improvement is noticeable.

Bellis (bellis perrenis), derived from the common daisy (also known as bruisewort, garden daisy or European daisy) is a good remedy to follow arnica. It acts directly on muscle tissue and the blood vessels to promote healing. Bellis has also been used to treat varicose veins and to ease post-surgery pain. Lower dosages (3c, 3x, 6x) are recommended for the treatment of bruises.

Hamamelis (hamamelis virginiana) has also been used to treat varicose veins and bleeding (such as from heavy periods in women). It is also recommended for injuries that result in bruising of the breast tissue. Hamamelis is derived from witch hazel, a plant used by Native Americans for its astringent and anti-inflammatory properties. Ruta and symphytum are also effective for dealing with bruises.

Homeopathic Treatments for Dislocations

The first course of action when dealing with a dislocation of a major joint is to seek medical attention. A dislocation may include injury to ligaments, tendons and nerves and should be immobilized. A dislocation to a major joint (shoulder, knee, elbow, jaw, ankle, etc.) is characterized by swelling, considerable pain and deformity to the injured area. Shock often accompanies this type of injury.

Arnica in mid- to high-range potencies can often assist with both the shock and immediate pain of the dislocation. Following relocation by an experienced medical practitioner, ruta can be administered in low- or mid-range potencies to deal with the trauma.

Bryonia (bryonia alba) is derived from the root of wild hops (also known as bryony or white bryony) and can be useful for swelling and pain resulting from slight movements of the relocated joint. It can be used in conjunction with arnica to address pain during the healing process.

Homeopathic Treatments for Fractures

A fracture may be indicated by pain and/or shock, inability to move the injured body part, swelling, bruising and deformation of the injured area. The injured area should be immobilized to prevent further damage until medical attention can be obtained. Arnica at mid-range potency can be taken every ten minutes to deal with the initial shock and pain of the fracture. It can then be taken every eight hours for up to four days. This may be followed by symphytum at a low potency every eight hours for two or three weeks.

Homeopathic Treatments for Golfer's Elbow and Tennis Elbow

Known to medical professionals as "medial epicondylitis" and "lateral epicondylitis" respectively, these arm injuries are not confined to the courts or the links. Golfer's elbow culminates in inflammation of the flexor and pronator muscles at the humerus, which is the bone of the upper arm. Tennis elbow occurs when the muscles of the forearm are strained at the point where they attach below the elbow. It can also result from an injury to the tendons on the outside of the elbow.

Arnica is the first homeopathic choice for muscle injuries. Low- to mid-potencies are suggested every half hour for the first two hours. Ruta can be taken three to four times a day for several days until the symptoms are noticeably improved. A dosage in the 6x, 30x to 30c range is suggested. Ruta and arnica can both be purchased as an ointment and applied topically to the injury.

Homeopathic Treatments for Sciatica

While sciatica is a disorder affecting the nervous system, it is often the result of an injury or degeneration from an injury. The sciatic nerve is the main nerve in the leg and is connected to nerves in both the pelvis and the spine. Sciatica is frequently felt in the buttock region and thigh, usually on one side of the body. Sciatica occurs when there is unusual pressure on the nerve. This may be the result of degeneration from osteoarthritis, a prolapsed vertebral disk or, in some cases, ankylosing spondylitis, an unusual autoimmune disease. Sciatic pain often flares up when an individual bends, sneezes or coughs.

When sciatic pain is worse from sitting and it is difficult to straighten the leg, Ammonium mur (ammonium chloratum) in low potencies such as 6c is recommended in half-hour doses for up to five hours. Common names for this mineral-derived remedy include sal ammoniac or ammonium chloride. Sciatica that is exacerbated by cold, damp weather resulting in numbness and weakness in the leg may be improved by colocynthis (cucumis colocynthis). Colocynthin is a substance found in a gourd known as bitter apple, bitter cucumber or colocynth. It causes severe cramps, and inflammation of the gastrointestinal tract if ingested. Hahnemann found it effective for treating these symptoms, as well as neuralgia. It can be used in the same potencies and dosages suggested for ammonium mur. Rhus tox (rhus toxicodendron) is used when sciatica is relieved by heat and movement, stretching the limbs and rubbing the painful area. Rhus tox comes from the leaves of poison ivy or poison oak. The dosages and potency suggested are the same as those above. Rhus tox can also be helpful in cases of tendonitis.

Homeopathic Treatments for Sprains

These injuries refer to damage to the ligaments. Ligaments are the fibrous, elastic connective tissues that surround joints. A sprain can refer to excessive stretching of the ligaments or, in the case of a severe sprain, the actual separation of the ligament from the joint.

Sprains are classified into three categories: first, second and third degree. First-degree sprains are the most common, resulting in tenderness and swelling around the injured joint. Second-degree sprains are identified with greater swelling and pain, as well as discoloration of the skin surrounding the joint. Joint movement may be limited with this injury. In addition to the symptoms above, a joint with a third-degree sprain will be unstable. For example, a person may not be able to support their weight on a severely sprained ankle. While first- and second-degree sprains are commonly addressed through anti-inflammatory medication, rest, ice, compression, elevation and heat, third-degree sprains should be evaluated and treated by a medical specialist.

In the case of homeopathic treatment of sprains, the homeopathic remedies often replace the anti-inflammatory medication. They can be used to combat pain, swelling and assist with the overall recovery. These remedies include arnica, bryonia or rhus tox, and ruta. As I have mentioned repeatedly, arnica is an excellent "first remedy" for most physical injuries, including sprains. A low- to mid-range potency every 30 minutes for up to two hours, followed by three doses daily will help combat the swelling and pain. If the injury is worsened by movement, I recommend low to medium potencies of bryonia in the same dosages as arnica. If the injury feels better when it is moved, I suggest using rhus tox in the same potencies and dosages as arnica. Ruta works best after the swelling and pain has subsided. It will promote healing of the ligaments and tendons and can be taken in 6x to 30x or 30c potencies every 30 minutes for up to four doses and three to four times daily until noticeable improvement takes place.

If an ankle is repeatedly sprained or easily sprained, ledum (ledum palustre) may be useful. This remedy is derived from wild rosemary (also known as marsh tea) and has been successfully used to address joints that are swollen, feel cold or make cracking noises when moved. Ledum may also been beneficial in cases of osteoarthritis.

6
STRENGTHENING, STRETCHING, BREATHING AND HEALING

Exercise is critical to your success in healing any injury. Immediately after an injury, you may need to rest first before embarking on an exercise program. However, it is important to begin therapeutic exercise as soon as possible. Start gradually and work up to doing more exercise. Remember, when it comes to injury, there is no such thing as "no pain, no gain." At the first sign of pain, stop what you're doing since you may add insult to injury. Prior to starting any new exercise program, particularly those sustained after an injury, it is important to check with your doctor.

The many benefits of exercise include:

- increased energy
- reduced stress
- burned fat
- improved metabolism
- greater bone mass
- increased oxygen to tissues and organs
- muscle toning and strengthening
- improved posture
- improved lung capacity
- greater flexibility
- stronger joints
- better-balanced spine and hips
- increased body awareness
- improved left- and right- brain hemisphere integration

- calmer mind
- greater relaxation
- increased self-confidence
- weight loss or gain (as needed)

However, not all types of exercise offer all of the above benefits. As well, these are just some of the benefits of exercise. There are also unique benefits to particular forms of exercise.

One of the main reasons people sustain injuries is their lack of muscular strength or imbalanced muscular strength. Exercise is essential for both men and women, although research still shows that women tend to exercise less than men. This ratio is slowly becoming more balanced. Women lose about one-third of their muscle mass between the ages of 35 and 80. Loss of muscle mass makes every task harder and requires more energy. As you read in chapter 1, exercise is also integral to building healthy bone mass. By some estimates, a ten-minute brisk walk will also provide one to two hours worth of increased energy.

There are many types of exercise, many of which are helpful for healing injuries. Some excellent forms of exercise that offer many of the benefits just mentioned and are suitable for your injury-healing program include:

- walking
- qigong
- yoga
- pilates
- strength training
- breathing exercises

Walking

Consider some of the following advantages of walking to help you heal your injuries:

- reduced risk of cancer, heart disease, and stroke
- very low injury risk
- reduced risk of diabetes by improving your body's ability to use insulin
- help in preventing osteoporosis by strengthening your bones
- potential weight loss
- improved sleep
- reduced stress and depression
- reduced PMS and menopausal symptoms

- reduced risk of injury (Fifty percent of all runners, recreational or competitive, develop injuries such as knee and hip problems, stress fractures, shin splints, and lower back problems. Walking is much easier on the body.)

Walking to improve your fitness status should be faster than a stroll. When strolling it takes about eight minutes to complete one kilometer (km). Walking should take five to six minutes to complete 1 km. Begin gradually after your injury and eventually work up to that pace. Be aware of your posture when walking. Hold your body tall and erect, with your head up and chin pulled back. Let go of any tension in your neck and shoulders and pull in your abdomen and buttocks to lengthen and straighten your spine.

Qigong

Qigong (pronounced "chee-gung") is an integrated mind-body healing technique that has been practiced in China for thousands of years and is gaining popularity in the West. "Qi" is the Chinese word for "life energy" and "gong" can be translated as "work" or "benefits acquired through perseverance and practice," according to Ken Cohen, one of the foremost Western practitioners of qigong. It is a holistic system of self-healing exercises and meditation, focusing primarily on breathing techniques, movement, self-massage and posture.

Qigong helps to:

1. improve energy circulation through the entire body;
2. replace impure or diseased "qi" with pure, healing "qi"; and
3. improve overall health and well-being.

I find qigong an excellent form of exercise for anyone, but even people who have suffered very serious injuries can benefit from this gentle but powerful activity. Do not be fooled by how easy it appears, qigong offers countless healing benefits that make it a worthy pursuit.

There are two main types of qigong: 1) active or dynamic and 2) tranquil or passive. Active is the more commonly seen type, involving full or partial body movements in a series of postures, held or repeated for different lengths of time. Passive qigong is more like meditation, with a specific focus on controlling the qi through mental concentration and visualization while the body is still. In short, active qigong is exercise, passive qigong is meditation. Anyone can practice qigong, including young children and elderly people, people with no health problems or people with serious disabilities. It can be practiced standing, sitting or lying. Both forms are effective for healing injuries.

Consider the following study, cited in a report called "Effects of Qigong on Preventing Stroke and Alleviating the Multiple Cerebro-Cardiovascular Risk Factors - Follow-up Report on 242 Hypertensive Cases for 30 Years," conducted at the Shanghai Institute of Hypertension (at the Shanghai Second Medical University) on hypertension (high blood pressure) and related conditions. Participants were divided into two groups: 122 in the qigong group, 120 in the non-practitioner control group. All subjects took standard hypertensive medications and were monitored for 30 years. By the end of the 30 years, 47.76 percent of the subjects in the control group had died. In the qigong group 25.41 percent had died. The incidence of stroke in the control group was 40.83 percent. The incidence of stroke in the qigong group was 20.49 percent. The incidence of death due to stroke in the control group was 32.50 percent. The incidence of death due to stroke in the qigong group was 15.57 percent. Forty of the subjects were examined with ultrasound and the qigong subjects were found to have stronger heart muscles and better left ventricle function.

If other health concerns prevent you from following most forms of exercise, try qigong. You can join a class or follow along with a video. I have listed some of my favourite qigong exercise videos in the Resources section of this book.

Yoga

Yoga comes from the Sanskrit word "yug," which means, "to join together." Yoga is more than just stretching. Yoga also advocates a holistic approach to healthful living through ethical practice, physical exercises (known as "asanas"), breathing exercises (known as "pranayama") and meditation training.

Asanas, or stretching exercises, are designed to develop maximum flexibility and strength in the skeletal, muscular and nervous systems, with a special emphasis on a strong and supple spine. The exercises also serve to massage internal organs, improve circulation and increase oxygen and its distribution throughout the body and the brain at the cellular level. Yoga stretches and relaxes the body, calms the mind and emotions, and aids recovery from all forms of accumulated stress.

Yoga is therapeutic for people healing from injuries and studies show that it brings the following benefits:

1. reduces muscular tension and blood pressure;
2. improves oxygen intake, circulation, digestion and elimination;
3. regulates metabolism and the working of all the glands and organs; and
4. enhances the function of the nervous system for increased calmness and energy.

Some of the exercises suggested below are taken from yoga. I encourage you to follow them, but consider joining a yoga class or following along with a video as well. I have also included some of my favorite yoga exercises videos in the Resources section of this book.

Pilates

Named after its founder, Joseph Pilates, pilates is a unique combination of exercises to be performed in a specific order. By following this order of exercises, you're able to balance your body's structure, strengthen muscles, and lengthen your body. Pilates was designed specifically for healing from injuries, making it a perfect form of exercise as part of this program. Some of the exercises can be rather intense, so consult a doctor before undertaking them.

Joseph Pilates (born 1880 in Germany) studied human physiology and ways to improve it (modern research has since confirmed his insights). He developed a practice in New York helping athletes recover from injuries. The main premise of pilates is that it relies on building up your "powerhouse"—abdominal, lower back, buttock, and inner thigh muscles. In turn, these muscles help realign your spine and the rest of your body, helping it to heal from injuries and making it less prone to further injury.

Pilates brings the following benefits:

1. helps improve flexibility;
2. realigns the body;
3. improves mental alertness;
4. improves blood supply throughout the body;
5. decreases stress and tension;
6. improves breathing capacity; and
7. improves body shape and posture.

Maximum benefit comes from doing pilates exercises four times per week, although you will still reap many rewards if doing less. Consider joining a pilates class or following along with a video. I have included one of my favorite Pilates videos in the Resources section of this book.

The Role of Posture in Healing Injuries

Before beginning any stretching or strengthening program, we must first look at the role of posture in healing injuries. Most people have poor posture: we may slouch when we sit, hunch when we walk or stand, lean our necks forward, and tilt our feet inward or outward. While we may not have noticed the toll that poor posture takes on our health when we are well, it becomes essential to immediately pay attention and correct poor postural patterns when an injury occurs.

The negative fallout of poor posture includes:

- tension along the length of the spine, resulting in pain in the neck, shoulders, back, hips and legs;
- headaches and restrictive breathing;
- reduced circulation of blood and oxygen to alleviate inflammation and tension; and
- decreased blood and oxygen to organs and glands.

Two occupational therapists in New York City, Jane Gatanis and Alyssa Frey, have developed a powerful pain reduction program. Part of this program addresses incorrect posture. Their body-alignment exercise takes less than a minute to perform and helps align posture and deepen your breathing. With repeated use it will make you more aware of the various parts of your body, how your body feels, and make you feel more in control of the pain and tension. They recommend beginning by practising the exercise five times per day for the first two weeks and then three times per day afterward. It can be done almost anywhere, even waiting in line at the bank. If you're able to stand, here's how to perform this simple exercise:

- Stand with your feet firmly planted, about six inches apart. Keep your ankles parallel to each other and your slightly-bent knees facing forward. Try to keep your weight evenly distributed on your feet. Visualize that your big toe, little toe and heel are a stool that bears your weight evenly.

- With your arms at your sides, position your hands with your palms facing forward, allowing your chest to be more open.
- Using your lower abdominal muscles, gently pull your belly upward and inward. Your abdomen should only slightly flatten. Do not shift the position of your back unnaturally. Hold for five to ten seconds, breathing normally.
- Drop your shoulders downward and toward the back and lift your chest slightly.
- Visualize your head floating over your spine. Move your chin slightly back toward your neck and chest.
- Breathe in deeply to the count of five and exhale to the count of five. As you inhale, relax your upper abdominal muscles so the lower parts of your lungs fill with fresh air.

Most pain, even when caused by injuries, has an emotional component. You may find yourself in stressful situations and notice that you pull your shoulders up, tense your neck, sit more slouched, and/or cross your arms or legs. The end result is more pain. Some pain experts, including Jane Gatanis and Alyssa Frey, who in their occupational therapy practice have relieved people of even the most stubborn pain, believe that 95 percent of pain has an emotional component. Russel Portenoy, M.D., Chairman of the Department of Pain Medicine and Palliative Care at Beth Israel Medical Center and a leading expert on pain, states that there is more scientific evidence that mind-body approaches can be useful for pain than there is for most OTC and prescription pain medications.

For the best results it is essential in any injury-healing program to incorporate mind-body therapies with more traditional rehabilitative techniques. Acupressure is a powerful mind-body therapy so it is critical to use the techniques you will learn in the next chapter.

When considering the types of exercises you wish to include in your Eight-Week Injury-Healing Program, there are four forms of exercise to consider. I recommend that you include all four types on a regular basis. They are:

- stretching (incorporating the exercises mentioned next);
- strengthening (involving weight or resistance training, using free weights, equipment found in a health club, a Universal weight machine, pulleys, bands or rubber tubing);
- cardiovascular (any exercise that gets your heart rate up, including brisk walking, jogging, elliptical training, or other aerobic activity); and

- breathing (an excellent way to center your mind and clear it from the clutter of the day as well as to bring oxygen to all the cells of your body. I include one breathing exercise below but qigong incorporates many breathing exercises that are worth pursuing as well).

Exercises for the Neck

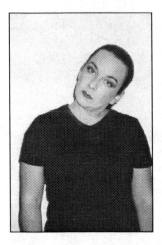

Side Bend

Relax your shoulders. Facing forward, slowly drop your ear toward your shoulder without raising your shoulder. Hold for ten seconds. Repeat on both sides.

Forward Bend

Relax your shoulders. Facing forward, slowly drop your chin down toward your chest. Hold for ten seconds.

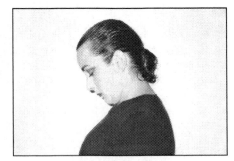

Head Turn

Relax your shoulders. Pull your chin back. Slowly turn your head to the left. Hold for ten seconds. Then return your head to face forward. Repeat with the right side.

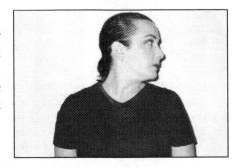

Exercises for the Back

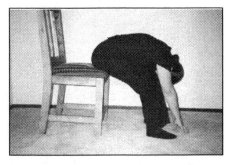

Sitting Forward Bend

Sitting on the edge of a chair with your feet placed firmly and wide apart on the floor, slowly lean forward and drop your hands to the floor, keeping your head and arms positioned between your knees. Keep your movement very slow and gentle. Hold the position for ten seconds.

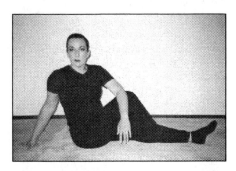

Sitting Spinal Twist

Sitting with your legs out-stretched on the floor, place your right leg over your left leg, keeping the right leg bent but the sole of the foot flat on the floor. Keep your back straight and your chin pulled back. Place your left elbow on the outside of your right knee and your right hand on the floor behind you. Breathe in and out, feeling your spine lengthen and your muscles stretch. Repeat on the opposite side.

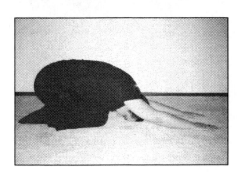

Lat Stretch

Kneeling on all fours on the floor, extend your arms straight out in front of you. Feel the stretch in your back muscles. Hold for ten seconds, continuing to breathe.

Cat Stretch

Kneel on all fours on a mat with your hands directly in front of your shoulders and your knees directly under your hips. Keep your back straight. Then, gently arch your back upward toward the ceiling, similar to a cat. Drop your head down and pull your pelvis in. Hold for twenty seconds then release.

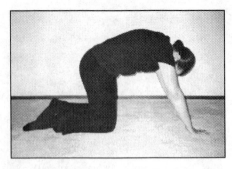

Knee Cradling

Lie on your back on a mat on the floor. Pull your knees to your chest and clasp them with your hands. Keeping your whole body as relaxed as possible, slowly pull your knees toward your chest. Hold for ten seconds and then release.

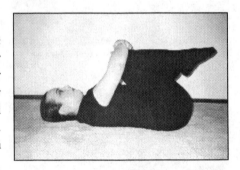

Bottom Raise

Lie on your back with your knees bent and feet flat on the floor, keeping your arms at your sides. Slowly lift your buttocks off the floor and hold as long as you are comfortable. Slowly drop your buttocks back to the floor.

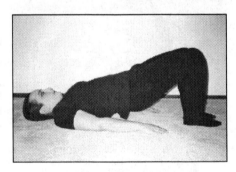

Exercises for the Hips

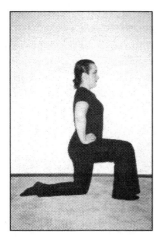

Hip Flexor Stretch

Kneel in an upright position. Keep your spine tall and straight. Pull your chin back. Look straight ahead. Bend your right knee and place your foot on the floor straight ahead of your right hip. Hold this pose for ten seconds, then switch legs and hold for ten seconds on the other side.

Pelvic Tilt

Lie on your back with your knees bent and your feet flat on the floor. Tighten the muscles in your abdomen and buttocks and press your low back into the floor. This should tilt your pelvis forward and up slightly. Relax your muscles and repeat ten times.

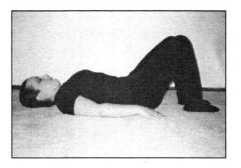

Exercises for the Knees

Quadriceps Stretch

Using the back of a chair for balance, stand with your spine tall and erect and your chin back. Bend your left leg and gradually pull your left foot toward your buttocks. Hold for ten seconds and change sides. Repeat. Make sure you keep the knee of the supporting leg slightly bent. Never lock your knees in a straightened position.

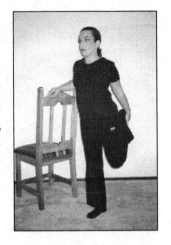

Hamstring Stretch

Stand with one foot in front of the other. Lean forward and bend the back knee, resting your hands on the bent knee. Bring your weight back and lift the front foot so it rests on the back of your heel. You should feel a stretch in the back of the leg. Hold this position for ten seconds. Repeat on the other side.

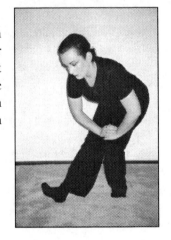

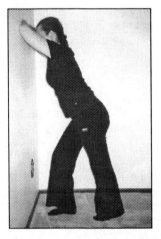

Calf Stretch

Stand facing a wall. Rest your arms on the wall and your face on your arms. Keep your right leg close to the wall with your left leg back. Slowly press your left heel toward the floor. You should feel a stretch in your calf muscle. Repeat on the other side.

Exercises for the Shoulders

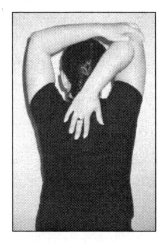

Triceps Stretch

Stand with your spine straight and tall. Lift one arm above your head and touch your back with that hand. Gently push the elbow backward with the opposite hand. Feel the stretch in your upper arm. Hold for ten seconds. Repeat on the other side.

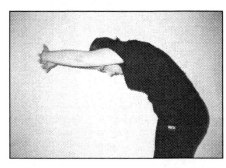

Upper Back Stretch

Clasp your hands in front of you and extend them forward. Do not lock your elbows. Keep them bent slightly. Round your shoulders, drop your head and feel the stretch across your upper back and shoulder area. Hold for ten seconds.

Chest Stretch

Stand with your spine straight and tall. Clasp your hands behind you with your knuckles out. Squeeze your shoulder blades together and feel the stretch in your chest. Hold for ten seconds.

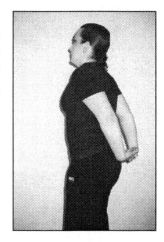

Shoulder Rolls

Stand with your spine straight and tall. Relax your shoulders. Slowly roll both shoulders in circles, feeling them loosen.

Shoulder Shrugs

Stand with your spine straight and tall. Relax your shoulders. Slowly bring your shoulders up toward your ears and then slowly drop back down again.

Breathing Exercises

I find doing the following simple breathing exercise throughout each day to be very beneficial, particularly to increase oxygen and improve energy flow in the body and thereby aid healing:

- Take several deep breaths, focusing on your breath's natural rhythm.
- Begin breathing into your solar plexus area, visualizing it becoming warm and relaxed.
- Continue breathing in and out into the solar plexus area for at least five minutes.

Exercise does not have to be difficult or tedious to be effective. It is important to enjoy whatever exercise you do. You will reap greater benefits that way. I suggest you add music and variety to your exercise to ensure that it is fun as well.

7
ACUPRESSURE FOR HEALING

Imagine being struck by an arrow in an ancient battle, recovering from the wound only to discover that your lifelong chest pains and breathing difficulties also disappeared. That is the legend behind the formation of acupuncture. Wounded soldiers were believed to have experienced the sudden healing of afflictions (that existed prior to battle) alongside the recovery of the arrow wound.

Tradition also states that acupuncture formed out of a dialogue between the Chinese ruler, Huang Di (the "Yellow Emperor") and his Prime Minister, Chi Po. No one knows exactly how this ancient healing art was first discovered, but it has stood the test of time, existing for at least five thousand years because it is remarkably effective for healing and pain reduction. Slight variations of it developed independently in China and India and among the ancient Aztecs. Compare this lengthy history to "modern medicine," which has been around for only 100 years or so.

How Acupuncture Works

Thousands of research studies have proven the healing effects of needling the body in specific locations known as "points" or "acupoints" but potentially millions of people have experienced the proof that acupuncture works by witnessing improvements in their symptoms. For those in need of scientific proof, engineers developed instruments called "acupunctuscopes" that prove the existence of the acupuncture points by reading the electrical frequency on the surface of the skin. Changes in electrical frequency occur in the exact location of the points on the body based on ancient texts and drawings.

These points exist in the body in connected lines known as "meridians" or "channels." While many studies had proved the existence of the acupuncture points, until recently scientists still doubted that they were connected.

Over a decade ago, French scientists went to work to prove or disprove the meridian theory. Taking two groups of people, they injected them with radioactive dye. One group was injected with dye in the exact location of the acupuncture points. Participants in the other group were injected in bogus points. The movement of the dye was monitored. Researchers were shocked to discover that where the dye had been injected into real acupuncture points, it flowed in lines in the positions of the meridians recorded by the Chinese millenia ago. Where the dye was injected into bogus points, the dye merely dispersed, without following any lines at all. Other studies have also confirmed the existence of meridians in the body.

Even the World Health Organization endorses acupuncture by publishing a list of dozens of illnesses that acupuncture effectively treats, including: headaches and migraines, osteoarthritis, bursitis, tendonitis, sciatica and other musculoskeletal disorders, neurological disorders, and countless others.

Essentially, the meridians are energy pathways in the body that when flowing properly, ensure health and vitality. However, when a blockage occurs (which can be caused by any number of things including stress, physical injuries, emotional traumas, allergies, poor nutrition, etc.) the flow of energy is disrupted and this disruption can cause a multitude of symptoms including pain, inflammation, and virtually any health problem. Energy meridians are similar to a river. If a tree falls in the river, it may disrupt the flow of water through the river and may even affect any tributaries that get their flow of water from the river. A blockage is comparable to the tree, disrupting the proper energy flow throughout the body. The acupressure points are locations along the energy lines where the energy surfaces in the body. These are the locations that the Chinese (and other cultures) documented over five thousand years ago, and whose existence recent research has confirmed. These points have a higher electrical frequency and respond very well to touch applied in the form of pressure or massage.

In China, acupuncture is practiced widely in hospitals and medical clinics. In the West, however, it has taken longer to catch on. Perhaps this is due to our experiences with needles, which we associate with large, thick instruments used for drawing blood or delivering vaccinations—the kind that make you jump out of your chair from discomfort or fear. Unlike these needles, acupuncture needles are quite fine, much thinner than a pin in fact.

So, how can this knowledge help you? You can take advantage of it in the healing of your injuries in two ways: 1) by visiting a skilled acupuncturist on a regular basis; and/or 2) by applying a form of modified acupuncture known as acupressure yourself. Acupressure uses simple finger pressure to alleviate blockages in the body, without the use of needles. Both techniques are effective. Typically, acupuncture works on a deeper healing level, but acupressure can produce similar results with regular use.

The Acupressure and Pain Connection

Using acupressure you can alleviate pain and speed the healing of your injuries. There are many reasons why acupuncture and acupressure work. One of the ways is that the sensation of pressure travels the same route to the brain as pain does.

Pain does not only occur in localized areas. It travels by way of the spinal cord and nervous system, thereby sending pain messages to the brain. Many sensations travel the same pathway as pain. In fact, like on a highway system, numerous sensations travel the same road. The speed of the sensation determines how quickly the message gets to the brain. This gives us a clue as to how to control pain. Pain actually travels this pathway quite slowly. Dull pain travels at approximately one-half mile to two miles per second. Sharp or burning pain travels at approximately five to 30 miles per second. Non-painful touch such as acupressure or massage travels at 35 to 75 miles per second.

The structure in the spine, through which these sensations travel, is known as the dorsal horn. Imagine this process of pain traveling through your body as similar to a sprint race in which runners are competing to grab a flag at the end. The person who grabs the flag first is the winner. Of course, the fastest runner will grab the flag and win. Similarly, if two kinds of sensations enter the dorsal horn in the spine at the same time, the fastest one will win.

You may have noticed that when many people get injured they grab the injured area immediately. This is an instinctive reaction and one that works on the premise that pressure travels faster than pain and can often cut off the pain response from the brain, thereby providing relief.

Massage works similarly. If you've ever noticed that massage helps alleviate pain (even if another area other than the injured area is massaged) it is because of this pathway by which sensation travels in the body. Again, massage sensations travel significantly faster than pain.

Topical pain creams or lotions that create a burning sensation have the same effect. Because they create a burning sensation that travels between five to 30 miles per second, it can, literally, beat pain to the brain, thereby lessening the feeling of pain. If you choose this approach, select a natural cream, gel or lotion that is devoid of harmful chemicals. You may need to search for one at a health food store. One that contains a compound called capsaicin (derived from hot peppers) tends to have pain-reducing and healing effects.

In this chapter, I am going to share some simple acupressure massage techniques that you can do yourself or you can enlist the help of another person. Based on the practice of acupuncture, acupressure uses finger pressure instead of needles to unblock the flow of energy that runs along the energy lines known as meridians.

In Chinese medicine, disease or pain is the result of a blockage of invisible energy that flows (although some gifted people can see this energy) along lines throughout the body, most of which connect with organs and organ systems. When this energy travels smoothly we experience a state of perfect health and energy. When the energy is disrupted, it causes many symptoms, including pain, inflammation, fatigue, headaches, and countless others. In the case of injuries, the injury typically disrupts the energy flow through the body, causing any number of health concerns.

Using simple acupressure techniques combined with the dietary and lifestyle suggestions in this book, you can promote healing of your injuries and experience relief from pain. Acupressure is effective in helping inflamed muscles and tendons heal as well as healing joint injuries.

Do It Yourself Acupressure

There are hundreds of acupressure points on the body. It is not essential to know all of the points to achieve pain relief or healing of your injuries since there are some major ones that are helpful for various types of injuries. Some points are in the area of the pain, while others are not. While proponents of acupressure often espouse specific approaches to pressing or rubbing the points, you can get great results from doing what feels right for you and not getting caught up in theory. You can either hold the points firmly or rub them in small circles, either clockwise or counter-clockwise, whichever feels best to you.

Please be patient. It may take some time while holding or massaging the points for the best results. But, the effort will be worth it. If you cannot press the points yourself, enlist the help of someone else to do it for you.

I have included some simple acupressure procedures for you to use in your Injury-Healing Program. Try to do the ones that are applicable to your injuries several times a day and stick with it for at least a month, although you will probably see results much faster. Just because the pain or other symptoms are gone does not mean the underlying energy blockage is adequately addressed. It may take longer to completely eliminate the energy blockage, but the result of doing so will be more complete healing that lasts longer.

I recommend that you avoid using massage oils or lotions when rubbing the points, as these will typically make your skin too slippery to hold the point for any length of time. In fact, you can be fully clothed while doing acupressure, making it easy to do anywhere. Some of the points are easily accessible and allow you to rub them in line at the grocery store, on a bus ride or in the car (as a passenger of course), or while watching television. If it is difficult for you to use your thumb or fingers to rub the points, you can also use your knuckle.

Avoid getting stressed about whether you're finding the point precisely. Sometimes, there will be some discomfort at the site of the point, while other times there won't be any noticeable sensation.

Many of the points are located on both sides of the body. Points along the "Ren" and "Du" channels, however, are not. Instead, these points run along the center line of the body. All the other points can be rubbed on both sides of the body. As difficult as it might be for some people to believe, if you cannot rub the point on the injured side of the body, rubbing the point on the other side of the body will still produce healing results and a lessening of pain.

If you do not see your particular problem among the acupressure treatments I have listed in the following section, choose the one that is closest to your problem. Where the injury is linked with a joint, it is an appropriate therapy for joint injuries as well as injuries to the muscles, tendons, ligaments, and other soft tissue in the surrounding area as well. For example, the acupressure listed under "Knee Injuries" can be used for injuries of the knee joint but also for muscle tears, damaged ligaments, or other injuries in the knee area.

For your convenience I have included with each injury the name of the point to hold, where it is located and the organ meridian the point is linked to. The points to hold are the same for many of the injuries so in some cases you will be reading the same descriptions of acupressure points over again. I felt it was better to repeat these descriptions rather than ask you to flip back and forth to an introductory description.

When trying to locate an acupressure point a general rule of thumb is, if you find a point on your body that feels sore, gently apply pressure. You may have discovered an energy blockage. Pressing on the area will help to disperse any blockages you might have. Do not be overly aggressive while pressing the area or you may cause bruising.

Do not be surprised if some of the points I am recommending are not even close to the location of the injury. In Chinese medicine, some of the best points for healing injuries are located somewhere totally different on the body. Yet, they are proven to be effective for healing and have been in use for thousands of years.

If you are pregnant, you should avoid using some points, namely LI4, and St 36. While there are other points to avoid during pregnancy, they are not relevant to injury healing and I have, therefore, not presented them. Avoid using acupressure during the first and last trimester of pregnancy as well. Pregnant or not, if you are uncertain as to whether to use acupressure or whether acupressure will negatively impact your injuries, please consult your doctor or an acupuncturist first.

Acupressure may look difficult at first but it is really quite simple. With practice you will find that it becomes easier. Soon, you will be reaching for the exact points at the first sign of pain. I urge you to take the initial time to become familiar with using acupressure since it is such a powerful healing modality.

In the section below I have included some of the best acupressure points for healing various injuries. They are categorized by location of the injury as this is more important than the name or type of injury for the purpose of acupressure. Beside each point name is the channel or meridian on which the point sits.

Acupressure for Ankle Injuries

DU 20 (Du channel)

The Du channel is one of the two main channels to supply energy to all the other meridians. It runs along the spine and over the head to the lips. Du 20 is arguably the most powerful point on the body and is located on the top of the head about two-thirds of the way to the back of the head, directly in the middle if you drew an imaginary line from the chin over the nose, between the eyes and over the head. It is found in a slightly soft spot that is sometimes tender to touch.

LI 4 (large intestine meridian)

Located at the top of the crease when you push your thumb against your forefinger.

LI 11 (large intestine meridian)

Located on the top side of the elbow about halfway along the crease when bending the elbow joint.

UB 60 (urinary bladder meridian)

Located on the outside of the leg, behind the ankle protrusion.

K 3 (kidney meridian)

Located on the inside of the leg behind the ankle protrusion.

K 6 (kidney meridian)

Located on the inside of the leg below the ankle protrusion.

St 41 (stomach meridian)

Located on the front of the leg at the level of the ankle, directly centered.

GB 40 (gall bladder meridian)

Located on the top of the foot, just below the ankle and slightly toward the outside edge of the foot.

Sp 9 (spleen meridian)

Located on the inside edge of the knee, at the lowest level of the knee. Use this point if swelling is involved.

UB 11 (urinary bladder meridian)

Located about one inch away from the spine (on both sides) at the level of the top of the shoulders. Use this point especially if there is degeneration of the joint or bone.

Acupressure for Back Injuries, Back Pain and Spinal Injuries

With regard to back injuries or back pain, there is a wonderful exercise called the "spinal flush" developed by Donna Eden in her book, *Energy Medicine*. It involves enlisting the help of a partner. You can stand with your back to your partner or lay face down on a bed or couch. Starting with the base of the neck, ask your partner to rub (in a clockwise motion) each notch between the vertebrae, down to the base of the spine. If there is a particularly painful spot, ask your partner to rub that area a bit longer. The whole exercise takes about two minutes and can be done fully clothed.

Having a partner perform a spinal flush on you on a daily basis (or repeatedly throughout the day if possible) will help you heal from any spinal injuries or back pain. In addition to stimulating nerve endings along the spine, the exercise encourages white blood cells to go to the area that is being rubbed, thereby speeding healing. As well, the points along the spine correlate to many of the acupressure points along the "Du" channel. This is a critical channel in the body as it supplies energy to all the other channels, which then feed the organs and glands. Moving any stagnant energy in this channel can help healing occur throughout the body.

In addition to the spinal flush, you can perform acupressure to help with back pain or injuries. If you have trouble reaching these points, enlist the help of a partner to rub them. Here are some of the main points to use.

Du 20 (Du channel)

The Du channel is one of the two main channels to supply energy to all the other meridians. It runs along the spine and over the head to the lips. Du 20 is arguably the most powerful point on the body and is located on the top of the head about two-thirds of the way to the back of the head, directly in the middle if you drew an imaginary line from the chin over the nose, between the eyes and over the head. It is found in a slightly soft spot that is sometimes tender to touch.

Du 2

(Not linked to a specific organ, the Du channel supplies energy to all the meridians in the body.) Du 2 is located near the base of the spine between the buttocks.

UB 31 (urinary bladder meridian)

Located near the top of the hip region on the back about an inch on both sides of the spine.

LI 4 (large intestine meridian)

Located at the top of the crease when you push your thumb against your forefinger. This point is excellent for relieving pain.

UB 11 (urinary bladder meridian)

Located about one inch away from the spine (on both sides) at the level of the top of the shoulders. Use this point especially if there is degeneration in the spine.

UB 40 (urinary bladder meridian)

Located in the center of the crease on the back of the knee.

UB 60 (urinary bladder meridian)

Located on the outside of the leg, behind the ankle protrusion.

Sp 9 (spleen meridian)

Located on the inside edge of the knee, at the lowest level of the knee. Use this point if swelling is involved.

Du 26

(Not linked to an organ, the Du channel supplies energy to all the meridians in the body.) Du 26 is ocated on the upper lip just below the nose.

SI 3 (small intestine meridian)

Located one thumb-width up from the top outside knuckle of the hand (toward the wrist).

UB 62 (urinary bladder meridian)

Located just below the ankle bone on the little toe side of the foot.

St 44 (stomach meridian)

Located on the top of the foot between the second and third toes (count the big toe as one, etc.).

Acupressure for Chest Injuries

DU 20 (Du channel)

The Du channel is one of the two main channels to supply energy to all the other meridians. It runs along the spine and over the head to the lips. Du 20 is arguably the most powerful point on the body and is located on the top of the head about two-thirds of the way to the back of the head, directly in the middle if you drew an imaginary line from the chin over the nose, between the eyes and over the head. It is found in a slightly soft spot that is sometimes tender to touch.

LI 4 (large intestine meridian)

Located at the top of the crease when you push your thumb against your forefinger. This point is excellent for relieving pain.

SJ 8 (sanjiao meridian)

Located on the top of the forearm about one and a half hand-widths up from the wrist line.

Lu 1 (lung meridian)

Located on the front of the chest where it meets the shoulder joint.

St 18 (stomach meridian)

Located on the chest approximately one inch below the nipple.

GB 24 (gall bladder)

Located on bottom edge of the ribs directly below the nipple.

GB 34 (gall bladder meridian)

Located on the outside edge of the leg near the kneecap approximately two thumb-widths below the edge of the knee.

Sp 9 (spleen meridian)

Located on the inside edge of the knee, at the lowest level of the knee. Use this point if swelling is involved.

Acupressure for Elbow Injuries

There are four main acupressure points to press or rub if you are trying to speed healing or lessen pain caused by an elbow injury.

Du 20 (Du channel)

The Du channel is one of the two main channels to supply energy to all the other meridians. It runs along the spine and over the head to the lips. Du 20 is arguably the most powerful point on the body and is located on the top of the head about two-thirds of the way to the back of the head, directly in the middle if you drew an imaginary line from the chin over the nose, between the eyes and over the head. It is found in a slightly soft spot that is sometimes tender to touch.

SI 8 (small intestine meridian)

Located on the inside edge of the elbow joint.

LI 4 (large intestine meridian)

Located at the top of the crease when you push your thumb against your forefinger. This point is excellent for relieving pain.

LI 10 (large intestine meridian)

Located on the top side of the lower arm about an inch below the elbow crease.

LI 11 (large intestine meridian)

Located on the top side of the elbow about halfway along the crease when bending the elbow joint.

Lu 5 (lung meridian)

Located on the inside line at the elbow, slightly off-center toward the thumb-side edge of the arm.

P 3 (pericardium meridian)

Located on the inside line at the elbow, in the center.

H 3 (heart meridian)

Located on the inside line at the elbow, slightly off-center, toward the little finger-side edge of the arm.

SJ 5

(Not linked to a specific organ, this meridian, also called "Triple Warmer," is responsible for balance and homeostasis in the body.) SJ 5 is located on the top side of the forearm about two inches above the wrist in the center.

SJ 10

(Not linked to a specific organ, this meridian, also called "Triple Warmer," is responsible for balance and homeostasis in the body.) SJ 10 is located one thumb-width directly above the tip of the elbow toward the shoulder.

Sp 9 (spleen meridian)

Located on the inside edge of the knee, at the lowest level of the knee. Use this point if swelling is involved.

Acupressure for Finger Injuries

Du 20 (Du channel)

The Du channel is one of the two main channels to supply energy to all the other meridians. It runs along the spine and over the head to the lips. Du 20 is arguably the most powerful point on the body and is located on the top of the head about two-thirds of the way to the back of the head, directly in the middle if you drew an imaginary line from the chin over the nose, between the eyes and over the head. It is found in a slightly soft spot that is sometimes tender to touch.

LI 4 (large intestine meridian)

Located at the top of the crease when you push your thumb against your forefinger. This point is excellent for relieving pain.

Ex 28 (extra points)

Located in the space between the knuckles on the hand when you make a fist.

SI 3 (small intestine meridian)

Located one thumb-width up from the top outside knuckle of the hand (toward the wrist).

Sp 9 (spleen meridian)

Located on the inside edge of the knee, at the lowest level of the knee. Use this point if swelling is involved.

Acupressure for Foot Injuries

Du 20 (Du channel)

The Du channel is one of the two main channels to supply energy to all the other meridians. It runs along the spine and over the head to the lips. Du 20 is arguably the most powerful point on the body and is located on the top of the head about two-thirds of the way to the back of the head, directly in the middle if you drew an imaginary line from the chin over the nose, between the eyes and over the head. It is found in a slightly soft spot that is sometimes tender to touch.

K 1 (kidney meridian)

Located on the base of the ball of the foot. This point is found in a slight depression.

K 3 (kidney meridian)

Located on the inside of the leg behind the ankle protrusion.

LI 4 (large intestine meridian)

Located at the top of the crease when you push your thumb against your forefinger. This point is excellent for relieving pain.

St 44 (stomach meridian)

Located on the top of the foot between the second and third toes (count the big toe as one, etc.).

Sp 9 (spleen meridian)

Located on the inside edge of the knee, at the lowest level of the knee. Use this point if swelling is involved.

Acupressure for Headaches

Du 20 (Du channel)

The Du channel is one of the two main channels to supply energy to all the other meridians. It runs along the spine and over the head to the lips. Du 20 is arguably the most powerful point on the body and is located on the top of the head about two-thirds of the way to the back of the head, directly in the middle if you drew an imaginary line from the chin over the nose, between the eyes and over the head. It is found in a slightly soft spot that is sometimes tender to touch.

LI 4 (large intestine meridian)

Located at the top of the crease when you push your thumb against your forefinger. This point is excellent for relieving pain.

St 8 (stomach meridian)

Located about an inch behind the upper outside edge of the forehead.

GB 14 (gall bladder meridian)

Located at the upper outside edge of the forehead near the hairline.

Du 23

(Not linked to an organ, the Du channel supplies energy to all the meridians in the body.) Du 23 is located in the middle of the head about an inch above the start of the hairline above the forehead.

GB 1 (gall bladder meridian)

Located on the bone at the outer edge of the eye.

UB 1 (urinary bladder meridian)

Located on the inside edge of the eyebrow (toward the nose).

Du 26

(Not linked to an organ, the Du channel supplies energy to all the meridians in the body.)Du 26 is located on the upper lip just below the nose.

GB 20 (gall bladder meridian)

Located on the back of the neck where the skull meets the neck about an inch on both sides of the spine.

GB 41 (gall bladder meridian)

Located on the top of the foot toward the outside edge about an inch and a half above the fourth toe (the toe nearest the little toe).

Lu 7 (lung meridian)

Located on the inside of the arm, about an inch and a half above the wrist crease on the thumb side of the wrist.

SJ 5

(Not linked to a specific organ, this meridian, also called "Triple Warmer," is responsible for balance and homeostasis in the body.) SJ 5 is located on the top side of the forearm about two inches above the wrist in the center.

Sp 9 (spleen meridian)

Located on the inside edge of the knee, at the lowest level of the knee. Use this point if swelling is involved.

St 44 (stomach meridian)

Located on the top of the foot between the second and third toes (count the big toe as one, etc.).

Acupressure for Hip Injuries/Hip Pain

Du 20 (Du channel)

The Du channel is one of the two main channels to supply energy to all the other meridians. It runs along the spine and over the head to the lips. Du 20 is arguably the most powerful point on the body and is located on the top of the head about two-thirds of the way to the back of the head, directly in the middle if you drew an imaginary line from the chin over the nose, between the eyes and over the head. It is found in a slightly soft spot that is sometimes tender to touch.

LI 4 (large intestine meridian)

Located at the top of the crease when you push your thumb against your forefinger. This point is excellent for relieving pain.

GB 29 (gall bladder meridian)

Located about halfway between the outside edge of the waist and the hip bone on the back of the buttocks region.

GB 30 (gall bladder meridian)

Located on the side of the buttocks slightly toward the hip bone.

GB 34 (gall bladder meridian)

Located on the outside edge of the leg near the kneecap approximately two thumb-widths below the edge of the knee.

UB 32 (urinary bladder meridian)

Located approximately one inch on both sides of the spine, approximately one hand-width below the waist level.

UB 40 (urinary bladder meridian)

Located in the center of the crease on the back of the knee.

Sp 9 (spleen meridian)

Located on the inside edge of the knee, at the lowest level of the knee. Use this point if swelling is involved.

Acupressure for Knee Injuries

Du 20 (Du channel)

The Du channel is one of the two main channels to supply energy to all the other meridians. It runs along the spine and over the head to the lips. Du 20 is arguably the most powerful point on the body and is located on the top of the head about two-thirds of the way to the back of the head, directly in the middle if you drew an imaginary line from the chin over the nose, between the eyes and over the head. It is found in a slightly soft spot that is sometimes tender to touch.

LI 4 (large intestine meridian)

Located at the top of the crease when you push your thumb against your forefinger. This point is excellent for relieving pain.

St 36 (stomach meridian)

Located in the space where the two lower leg bones meet just below and to the outer edge of the kneecap.

GB 34 (gall bladder meridian)

Located on the outside edge of the leg near the kneecap approximately two thumb-widths below the edge of the knee.

UB 11 (urinary bladder meridian)

Located about one inch away from the spine (on both sides) at the level of the top of the shoulders. Use this point especially if there is degeneration of the joint or bone.

UB 60 (urinary bladder meridian)

Located on the outside of the leg, behind the ankle protrusion.

St 44 (stomach meridian)

Located on the top of the foot between the second and third toes (count the big toe as one, etc.).

Sp 9 (spleen meridian)

Located on the inside edge of the knee, at the lowest level of the knee. Use this point if swelling is involved.

Acupressure for Migraine Headaches

Migraines are a specific form of severe headache that are often accompanied by nausea, spots in front of the eyes, inability to tolerate light, impaired balance, vomiting, and diarrhea. I have heard many people refer to their headaches as "migraines," when they are in fact another form of headache. Be sure to get a diagnosis from your doctor since migraines can be potentially serious. If you do not have all or almost all of these symptoms, refer back to the "Headaches" section. For migraines use acupressure on the following:

Ren 12

(Not linked to an organ, the Ren channel supplies energy to all the meridians in the body.) Ren 12 is located in the middle of the abdomen about four finger-widths above the navel.

Du 20 (Du channel)

The Du channel is one of the two main channels to supply energy to all the other meridians. It runs along the spine and over the head to the lips. Du 20 is arguably the most powerful point on the body and is located on the top of the head about two-thirds of the way to the back of the head, directly in the middle if you drew an imaginary line from the chin over the nose, between the eyes and over the head. It is found in a slightly soft spot that is sometimes tender to touch.

Du 12

(Not linked to an organ, the Du channel supplies energy to all the meridians in the body.) Du 12 is located three vertebrae below the base of the neck (third thoracic vertebra).

St 44 (stomach meridian)

Located on the top of the foot between the second and third toes (count the big toe as one, etc.).

Acupressure for Neck Injuries

Du 20 (Du channel)

The Du channel is one of the two main channels to supply energy to all the other meridians. It runs along the spine and over the head to the lips. Du 20 is arguably the most powerful point on the body and is located on the top of the head about two-thirds of the way to the back of the head, directly in the middle if you drew an imaginary line from the chin over the nose, between the eyes and over the head. It is found in a slightly soft spot that is sometimes tender to touch.

Du 14 (Du channel)

Located along the spine in the notch between the vertebrae at the level where the neck and shoulders join.

LI 4 (large intestine meridian)

Located at the top of the crease when you push your thumb against your forefinger. This point is excellent for relieving pain.

SJ 5 (sanjiao meridian)

(Not linked to a particular organ, this meridian, also called the "Triple Warmer," is responsible for maintaining balance in the body.) SJ 5 is located on the top side of the forearm about two inches above the wrist in the center.

GB 20 (gall bladder meridian)

Located on the back of the neck where the skull meets the neck about an inch on both sides of the spine.

GB 21 (gall bladder meridian)

Located on the top of the shoulder about halfway between the outer edge of the shoulder joint and the neck.

Lu 7 (lung meridian)

Located on the inside of the wrist approximately one inch above the wrist line, toward the outer thumb edge.

GB 39 (gall bladder meridian)

Located on the outside edge of the lower leg approximately two inches above the top of the ankle.

UB 11 (urinary bladder meridian)

Located about one inch away from the spine (on both sides) at the level of the top of the shoulders. Use this point especially if there is degeneration of the joint or bone.

Sp 9 (spleen meridian)

Located on the inside edge of the knee, at the lowest level of the knee. Use this point if swelling is involved.

Acupressure for Shoulder Injuries

Du 20 (Du channel)

The Du channel is one of the two main channels to supply energy to all the other meridians. It runs along the spine and over the head to the lips. Du 20 is arguably the most powerful point on the body and is located on the top of the head about two-thirds of the way to the back of the head, directly in the middle if you drew an imaginary line from the chin over the nose, between the eyes and over the head. It is found in a slightly soft spot that is sometimes tender to touch.

LI 15 (large intestine meridian)

Located on the upper outer edge of the shoulder joint towards the back.

SI 9 (small intestine meridian)

Located on the back about two inches above the location where the arm meets the shoulder.

SI 14 (small intestine meridian)

Place your palm on your shoulder between the neck and the shoulder joint. Reach toward your back with your middle finger, which should be at approximately the location of SI 14.

St 38 (stomach meridian)

Located on the outside edge of the shinbone about halfway between the ankle and the knee. Do not let the distance of this point from the shoulder fool you. It is an effective point in Chinese medicine for shoulder injuries or pain.

SJ 14 (sanjiao meridian)

Located on the back of the shoulder joint in the depression approximately two inches below the top of the body.

LI 15 (large intestine meridian)

Located on the front of the shoulder joint approximately two and a half to three inches from the top of the body.

LI 4 (large intestine meridian)

Located at the top of the crease when you push your thumb against your forefinger. This point is excellent for relieving pain.

Sp 9 (spleen meridian)

Located on the inside edge of the knee, at the lowest level of the knee. Use this point if swelling is involved.

Acupressure for Wrist Injuries

Du 20 (Du channel)

The Du channel is one of the two main channels to supply energy to all the other meridians. It runs along the spine and over the head to the lips. Du 20 is arguably the most powerful point on the body and is located on the top of the head about two-thirds of the way to the back of the head, directly in the middle if you drew an imaginary line from the chin over the nose, between the eyes and over the head. It is found in a slightly soft spot that is sometimes tender to touch.

LI 4 (large intestine meridian)

Located at the top of the crease when you push your thumb against your forefinger. This point is excellent for relieving pain.

LI 11 (large intestine meridian)

Located on the top side of the elbow about halfway along the crease when bending the elbow joint.

P 7 (pericardium meridian)

Located on the inside of the wrist crease in the center.

H 7 (heart meridian)

Located on the inside of the wrist crease toward the little finger edge of the wrist.

Lu 9 (lung meridian)

Located on the inside of the wrist crease toward the thumb-side edge of the wrist.

St 44 (stomach meridian)

Located on the top of the foot between the second and third toes (count the big toe as one, etc.).

SJ 5

(Not linked to a specific organ, this meridian, also called "Triple Warmer," is responsible for balance and homeostasis in the body.) Located on the top side of the forearm about two inches above the wrist in the center.

Sp 9 (spleen meridian)

Located on the inside edge of the knee, at the lowest level of the knee. Use this point if swelling is involved.

Acupressure for Arthritis/Bursitis/Joint Inflammation

Follow the instructions above that pertain to the particular joint that is injured. In addition, add:

Sp 9 (spleen meridian)

Located on the inside edge of the knee, at the lowest level of the knee. Use this point if swelling is involved.

Acupressure for Fibromyalgia

Many people begin to have pain throughout their whole body after the onset of an injury or accident, where even being touched is uncomfortable. If you've been diagnosed with fibromyalgia, a rheumatic disorder that is characterized by achy muscular pain that most commonly affects the neck, shoulders, back of the head, upper chest, buttocks, and/or thighs, acupressure can be helpful in your recovery. Many people with fibromyalgia avoid massage types of therapies due to the pain they are experiencing, but acupressure can be very therapeutic. Just remember to be gentle while holding the points. Begin with the Spinal Flush described under "Back Injuries" above. This will help to improve energy flow throughout the body. There are numerous places on the body that are "tender points." Find these places on your body and gently press them, or ask a partner to help. These places include:

- Around the lower vertebra of the neck;
- At the insertion point of the second rib (from the top);
- Around the upper part of the thigh bone;
- In the middle of the knee joint;
- In the muscles connected to the base of the skull;
- In the muscles of the neck and upper back;
- In the muscles of the mid-back;
- On the side of the elbow; and
- In the upper and outer muscles of the buttocks.

In addition to these areas, also rub the Du 20 point (Du channel). The Du channel is one of the two main channels to supply energy to all the other meridians. It runs along the spine and over the head to the lips. Du 20 is arguably the most powerful point on the body and is located on the top of the head about two-thirds of the way to the back of the head, directly in the middle if you drew an imaginary line from the chin over the nose, between the eyes and over the head. It is found in a slightly soft spot that is sometimes tender to touch.

The key to effectiveness using acupressure is regularity. It is not adequate to do self-acupressure once per week. Daily treatments are ideal. Try to take the ten minutes or so per day to improve your pain and healing with this powerful modality.

Figure 7.1

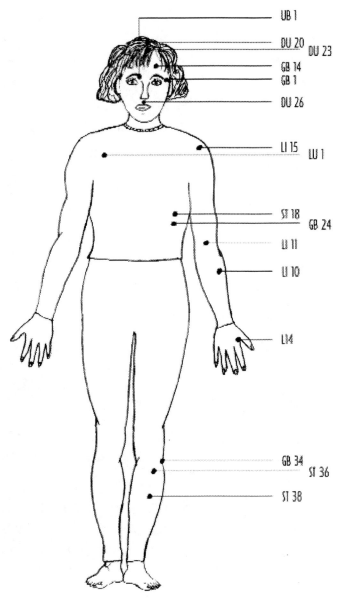

UB 1
DU 20
DU 23
GB 14
GB 1
DU 26
LI 15
LU 1
ST 18
GB 24
LI 11
LI 10
LI 4
GB 34
ST 36
ST 38

Figure 7.2

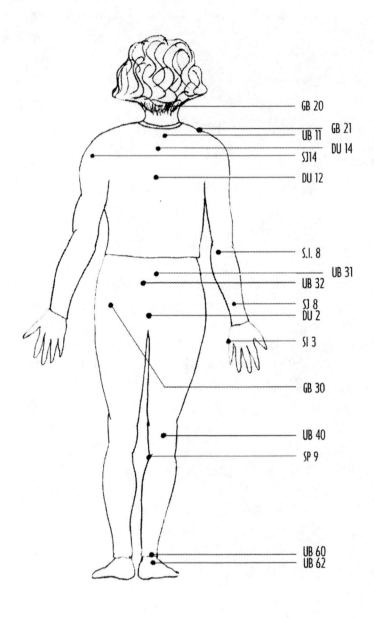

Figure 7.3

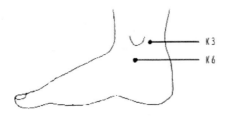

Figure 7.4

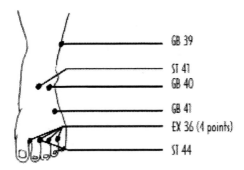

Figure 7.5

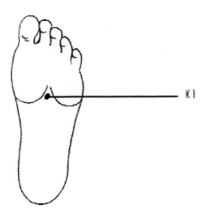

Figure 7.6. - Elbow (Inside)

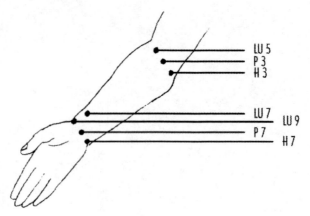

LU 5
P 3
H 3

LU 7
LU 9
P 7
H 7

Figure 7.7

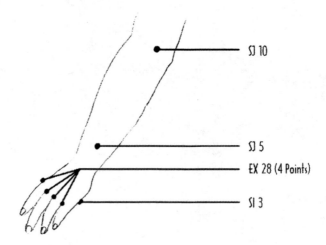

SJ 10

SJ 5
EX 28 (4 Points)
SI 3

8
NATURAL THERAPIES

There are many fabulous therapies that can be used to speed healing, improve healing results, or lessen symptoms along the way. Some of my favorites for healing injuries include: acupuncture, the Alexander technique, aromatherapy, Bach flower therapy, the Bowen technique, chiropractic, the cranio-sacral technique, detoxification therapy, energy medicine, Feldenkrais therapy, herbalism (Chinese, European or North American), homeopathy, lymphatic drainage, massage, naturopathy, nutritional therapy, osteopathy, quantum biofeedback, reiki, shiatsu, and Thai yoga massage.

Each discipline is quite extensive so I have briefly summarized each one in this chapter. The best healing results can be achieved by following the Eight-Week Injury-Healing Program outlined further on in this book while incorporating some of the natural therapies in this chapter.

Acupuncture

As I mentioned earlier, acupuncture is a powerful healing modality that should be considered for treating injuries because of its proven effectiveness. It is a highly respected healing modality that is many times older than "modern" medicine. Acupuncture is at least 5,000 years old. By other estimates, it may be 10,000 years old.

It works on several different premises, but the main one is the energy of the body, which acupuncturists refer to as "chi" or "qi" (both are pronounced "chee"). This energy, or life force, is found in the body, in air, water, food, and while it may be invisible, is proven to be integral to life.

In Chinese philosophy, there are dualistic streams of life force energy, called "yin" and "yang." To provide optimum health it is essential to balance these energies in the body. An injury can disrupt the natural flow of energy throughout the body, resulting in pain, inflammation, or other symptoms.

Acupuncturists use different methods of gathering information about your health in an effort to select the right acupuncture points for inserting needles. The most common ones include tongue diagnosis, pulse diagnosis, questioning you about your symptoms and what makes them better or worse, as well as other visual clues from your face or eyes.

The acupuncturist will then select which points he or she will use to bring balance back to the system and insert fine needles into those areas. Most people barely feel the insertion of these needles, which are much finer than a pin. Acupuncture is renowned for its effectiveness in relieving pain. In China, most hospitals do not use anesthesia drugs; instead, they rely on acupuncture anesthesia for major or minor surgeries or pain relief.

Many types of injuries or injury-related conditions have improved using acupuncture. Usually, the acupuncturist will recommend two or three sessions per week for the first three weeks. Afterward, he or she will determine the frequency of visits based on necessity and severity of the prevailing condition.

The Alexander Technique

The Australian actor Frederick Mathias Alexander created this technique at the turn of the century. He had chronic voice problems and went in search of a solution to save his voice and career. He frequently lost his voice while on stage and regained it later while resting. In an effort to discover why, he studied his body in the mirror, watching his posture during movements very closely. When he mimicked his acting roles he frequently noticed how the position of his head shifted, placing increasing levels of stress on his neck and his breathing. He could feel how his throat tightened and made attempts to correct the position of his head and body while he delivered his lines. He believed that by correcting negative postural and attitudinal patterns he could influence his health concerns. Because of the importance of correct posture in healing from injuries, the Alexander technique is an excellent choice of therapies.

The trained Alexander practitioner re-educates clients to become aware of correct and incorrect bodily positions while lying, sitting, standing, and walking. This enables clients to make conscious choices to improve their health. The added stress on the body resulting from poor posture often results in pain or injuries that won't heal adequately. The Alexander technique is an effective treatment for postural problems and an important component of healing injuries. It has worked well for rounded shoulders, stoops, over- or under-arched back, backaches, tight neck and throat, headaches, repetitive strain injuries like carpal tunnel syndrome, breathing and respiratory conditions, voice problems, arthritis, and many others.

The sessions take place while you are fully clothed. In a very gentle manner, the instructor will guide your posture in various positions. You will learn how to change harmful body positions into health-promoting ones that minimize the stress on your spine, muscles, nerves, and soft-tissue in the body.

Aromatherapy

Aromatherapy is the therapeutic use of natural oils from flowers, plants, trees, resins, and other elements in nature that have healing properties. It may involve inhaling the scent or rubbing the oil on part of the body. While the modern study of aromatherapy only started in the last century, aromatherapy is undoubtedly many thousands of years old. There is plenty of archaeological evidence to suggest that aromatherapy oils were regularly used in the ancient temples of Egypt, Greece and Rome.

Since that time there has been countless research at some of the world's leading universities on the effects of essential oils (potent plant extracts that contain the "essence" of the plant) on pain, inflammation, infection, depression, dementia, and many other symptoms.

Aromatherapy is often deemed to have mild effects due to the seemingly gentle nature of using the oils. This could not be further from the truth. When used correctly by a skilled aromatherapist, essential oils can have powerful results. Aromatherapy works in a number of ways, the main one being via the cells in the nose sending rapid messages to the brain, which results in the brain sending a quick message around the body, depending on the scent that was detected.

Each oil has unique therapeutic traits, usually many in a single oil. Each plant can produce more than one type of oil, for example, there are two types of essential oils derived from the orange tree: neroli oil from the blossoms and orange oil from the peel of the oranges.

Oils can be divided into one of three main classifications based on their general properties: uplifting, balancing, or calming. It is important to choose a very high quality oil since the therapeutic effects are greatly diminished in lesser oils. While there are many types of oils in the marketplace, few are produced to maintain the integrity of the plant. Avoid oils from some of the large bath and body product shops since these oils tend to be low quality. Also, avoid oils that are labeled "fragrance" oils, or "natural-like" oils since they're usually synthetic chemicals that offer no therapeutic value whatsoever.

A visit to a skilled aromatherapist who uses only the most natural, wild crafted or organic oils is a worthwhile investment to aid the healing of an injury. He or she can blend a suitable oil to help manage pain, inflammation, increase relaxation or improve energy levels and moods. Some oils have proven effects on infection as well.

Bach Flower Remedies

British medical doctor and bacteriologist Dr. Edward Bach founded a system of treating emotional imbalances using the "essence" of flowers. He carefully studied and developed remedies from wild flowers to work on mental fixations and emotions that may be producing harmful effects on the body.

Bach flower therapy is practiced by many homeopaths (see further on) and other natural health practitioners. The basic principle is simple. People with fearful, worried, or depressed mental states heal slower and less completely than do those with positive, cheerful, and hopeful states of mind.

Dr. Bach identified 38 remedies that can be used for virtually any combination of troublesome emotions. It is important to identify the remedy that most fits your mental/emotional patterns for the greatest success in using them.

Because injuries of any kind have an emotional component, I have included information about using Bach flower remedies, either with the help of a health practitioner who can help you select the most appropriate one(s) or for those people who would like to self-treat I have included a very basic overview of the flower remedies and the emotional states they best serve. Most health food stores sell Bach flower remedies. They come in small glass bottles with a dropper lid or as a throat spray. Simply take four drops under the tongue away from food or beverages.

Flower Remedies for Various Emotional States

Of all the flower remedies I mention next the rescue remedy is excellent for use immediately after any type of trauma or injury since it covers a cross-section of the most common emotional states following an accident.

The use of flower remedies is truly a skilled art as much as homeopathy is. Since everything on the planet has an energetic component to it (and one that physicists have been able to prove), Edward Bach, M.D., felt that this energy could be harnessed as a healing tool. Similar to homeopathy, minute amounts of plant energies (in this case in liquid drops) applied under the tongue cause a change in the energy of the person consuming them. Dr. Bach studied flowers, not only for their proven medicinal properties, but also for subtler, energetic properties and how they might affect health. He found substantial improvements in his patients' emotional well-being after dispensing the remedies he created from various flowers. He observed that a particular remedy had the greatest effect on a specific emotional pattern in people. You may find your particular emotional state (and the corresponding remedy) in the following list of negative emotions compiled by Lisha Simester in her book, *The Natural Health Bible*:

- Agrimony: suffers a lot internally, but keeps it hidden;
- Aspen: afraid of unknown things;
- Beech: arrogant, critical, and intolerant;
- Centaury: weak-willed, subservient, and easily used;
- Cerato: lacking in self-confidence, asks advice;
- Cherry plum: afraid of going crazy, losing control, or causing harm, violent temper;
- Chestnut bud: fails to learn from experience, repeats mistakes;
- Chicory: overly possessive, selfish and attention seeking;
- Clematis: absentminded, dreamy, and mentally escapist;
- Crab apple: self-dislike, feels unclean;
- Elm: feels temporary inadequacy;
- Gentian: depressed with known cause, easily discouraged;
- Gorse: depressed, all seems pointless;
- Heather: obsessed with own problems;
- Holly: jealous, suspicious, desiring revenge, full of hate;
- Honeysuckle: lives in the past;
- Hornbeam: procrastinates;
- Impatiens: impatient;
- Larch: depressed, feels inferior, expects to fail;
- Mimulus: afraid of known things;
- Mustard: deeply depressed without reason;
- Oak: grave, plodding, determined;
- Olive: mentally and physically exhausted;
- Pine: feels guilty, blames self;

- Red chestnut: afraid of others;
- Rescue remedy (a combination of cherry plum, clematis, impatiens, and Star of Bethlehem): used for shock, trauma, and external and internal first aid;
- Rock rose: feels terror, panic;
- Rock water: self-demanding, self-denial;
- Scleranthus: indecisive, mood swings;
- Star of Bethlehem: in shock;
- Sweet chestnut: despair, no hope left;
- Vervain: fanatical, tense, overenthusiastic;
- Vine: ambitious, tyrannical, demanding, unbending, power seeking;
- Walnut: the "link" breaker, for times of change;
- Water violet : reserve, pride, reliability;
- White chestnut: persistent thoughts and mental chatter;
- Wild oat: helps define goals;
- Wild rose: apathetic slacker, unambitious;
- Willow: bitter, resentful.

The Bowen Technique

The Bowen technique is a gentle therapy that involves a specific series of vibrational movements applied to muscles, tendons, and connective tissue. While it involves hands-on techniques, it is quite different from massage. It is beneficial for any stage of an injury but also valuable in the case of long-term pain as a result of an old injury. Developed by Tom Bowen, an Australian, in the 1950s, it is now a recognized therapy with widespread use around the world. The Bowen technique is useful for treating chronic or acute musculoskeletal pain and to help heal and regenerate tissues from injuries due to both sports and trauma.

Bowen is a form of gentle massage that targets specific muscles in the body to release any built up tension, thereby helping the body to align. It is quite relaxing but do not let that fool you. It is also quite powerful at releasing physical and emotional stress patterns that are stored in the body. Each Bowen session lasts approximately 45 minutes and, unlike most forms of massage, is performed with a client wearing light clothing.

Chiropractic

Chiropractic has come a long way since Daniel David Palmer first used it in 1895. Palmer first treated his office cleaner who had become deaf following a back injury. Palmer noted that some of the bones in the cleaner's spine had become misaligned. After manipulation of these bones, the cleaner's hearing was restored.

Palmer, who subsequently founded the Palmer School of Chiropractic, has this to say aboutchiropractic: "Displacement of any part of the skeletal frame may press against nerves which are channels of communication, intensifying or decreasing their carrying capacity, creating either too much or not enough functioning, an aberration known as disease."

That is the basic principle of chiropractic, which has since developed into many different forms, ranging from the more traditional manipulations using high velocity thrusts to gentler varieties such as "network chiropractic" that involve gentle strokes to lessen muscular tension. The aim of chiropractic is to correct disorders of the joints and muscles, particularly of the spine, by bringing the vertebrae back into alignment. Some chiropractors also work on the muscles, ligaments and tendons using various adjunct therapies.

While chiropractic has received some negative, arguably even sensational, media exposure in recent times, I still regard this form of therapy as highly beneficial to healing from injuries.

Chiropractic sessions vary in length, and may involve X-rays, massage, examination of the spine and other areas, manipulation of the joints while a patient is lying down, or a number of other procedures.

Cranio-Sacral Therapy

Cranio-sacral therapy is a gentle healing technique that involves light touch on the tiny joints of the skull, known as sutures. Founded by William Garner Sutherland, a trained osteopath in the early twentieth century, who was taught as part of his education that the bones of the skull were firmly fixed and immovable. He believed otherwise based on his experience. His theory was that, while the movements were only minute, a slight adjustment to the bones of the skull would often result in profound healing experiences for patients.

With additional experience, Sutherland learned that there are certain rhythms in the cranium that echo the fluctuation of cerebrospinal fluid (the liquid that bathes the tissues of the spinal cord and brain). Injuries or illnesses can result in less than optimal flow of this fluid (which is ten to 14 beats per minute). Using gentle manipulation of the head and sacrum (lower part of the spine), the pulse can be re-established and aid in healing the disease or disorder.

Modern cranio-sacral therapists are rarely doctors; usually, they receive training from the Upledger Institute, founded by Dr. John Upledger, an American osteopath.

The patient is most likely fully clothed during a cranio-sacral session unless the practitioner is also an osteopath who may want to observe the entire spine. With the patient in a prone position the practitioner gently manipulates the head and/or sacrum. The touch is so minimal that some people wonder if anything is being done. Keep in mind that the cerebrospinal pulse is so light that a delicate touch is required for adjustments. When it comes to therapy, particularly for injuries, gentler is almost always more effective. Usually treatments last between 30 minutes and one hour.

Detoxification

While it may sound odd to consider detoxification as a form of healing for an injury, it can be quite effective. Any number of toxins from the air, food, environment, soil, water, and other sources may enter our bodies. While our detoxification systems, like the liver, kidneys, lymph glands, bowels, and others are capable of lessening the effect of toxins on the body, at times the body's "toxic load" may become too great, creating an overall burden on the body and its healing mechanisms. Injuries that involve swelling and inflammation may place a further load on the body's detoxification systems. Cleansing the body of its waste products can help alleviate pain, inflammation, and promote healing.

There are some detoxification therapists who can help in this regard although in my experience, there are many people offering detoxification programs who are not well versed in this complex art and science. So, be cautious in choosing a practitioner.

There are many ways to detoxify, but one of the most effective ways is to follow the protocol listed in my Eight-Week Injury- Healing Program outlined in chapter 10 using cleansing foods and limiting intake of foods that stress the body.

Energy Medicine

As you already learned in the last chapter, your body (and all living things for that matter) consists of energy, which is an invisible, yet proven, force that enables us to live. There are many forms of energy in the human body: metabolic energy, bioelectrical energy, and biophotonic energy, to name a few. For the purpose of this book, I'll be referring to the subtle, or vital, bioenergy (also known as "subtle energy" or "magetic energy"). The two main forms of energy in the human body are: 1) the energy of "qi," discovered in China and based on the existence of meridians and channels throughout the organs, limbs, and around the whole body; and 2) the energy of "prana," discovered in India and premised on the existence of spirals of energy, also known as chakras, located along the spine and other places in the body. Both systems are valid and in fact work together to power our bodies.

Energy medicine is a broad category of therapies that utilize energy for the purpose of healing. Acupuncture and acupressure accomplish this by working on specific points along energy lines in the body to remove blockages that impede the flow of energy. Reiki works primarily on the chakras, but all forms of energy medicine focus on balancing the flow of energy in the body.

There is also a specific form of therapy called "energy medicine," which involves a variety of techniques to balance the body's energy systems, including touch, working on the aura of a person (this can be photographed using a specific form of photography known as Kirlian photography), or by exercises.

Because "energy medicine" as a discipline is lesser known, it may be more difficult to find a practitioner; however, it is worth the effort since it is quite a powerful therapy. Most "energy medicine" practitioners believe that healing at the energetic level precedes healing at a physical level, therefore, it is critical to work on transforming your body's energies to ensure full healing from an injury.

Sessions will vary from one practitioner to another. Some will ask you to sit, while others request that you lie on a padded table. Some therapists will use muscle testing to determine problems in the body, while others will not. Some practitioners will employ healing touch while others may work only in the aura. Similarly, some people will ask you to do energy-enhancing exercises while others will not. You will remain fully clothed.

Far-Infrared Sauna Therapy

Increasing one's body temperature has been used for millennia by cultures around the world to improve health and treat disease. Today, there are many tools employed to artificially raise body temperature, from heat lamps to wraps, quilts to hair dryers. The one common denominator among the best of these approaches is the use of far-infrared radiation (FIR) to create and deliver heat to the body. And, one of the best uses of FIR technology for health promotion is the sauna.

Clearly, the word "radiation" has negative connotations in modern society. We go out of our way to avoid anything that emits radiation or is "radioactive." However, there are many different forms of radiation. A nuclear bomb blast spreads atomic radiation that can be lethal. Ultraviolet radiation can damage the skin by causing burns. The most familiar example of this would be the harmful rays from the sun that penetrate the ozone layers and cause sunburns. In contrast, infrared radiation is what we often describe as "the healing warmth of the sun." It is radiant heat, which is a form of energy that heats objects directly, without having to heat the air in between. A classic example of this is being outside on a sunny day when a cloud suddenly obscures the sun. In that short time, the air temperature has not changed but there is a noticeable chill until the cloud passes and the sun is visible again. This is the principle behind radiant heat, or infrared radiation.

Infrared radiation is measured as light along the electromagnetic spectrum. It falls just below ("infra") the red light segment. It is not visible to the human eye. Infrared light penetrates beyond the skin level and is absorbed by the cells. In contrast, visible light simply bounces off the skin. Near-infrared light is absorbed at the skin level and will cause the surface skin temperature to increase slightly. Far-infrared light penetrates an estimated four centimeters, working energetically at the cellular level to increase metabolism and blood circulation, as well as elevating the core body temperature—all of which can promote healing of injuries and detoxification of the body. Some FIR saunas adopt this process through ceramic infrared heaters to bring additional health benefits to the traditional sauna experience.

One of the clearest advantages of FIR saunas is the sweat-to-temperature ratio. The energy emitted by FIR saunas will result in a "sweat volume" two to three times greater than a conventional steam sauna and do so at a much lower temperature. FIR saunas operate in the 110° to 130° F range while conventional steam saunas will reach temperatures in the 180° to 235° F range. Many individuals find these latter temperatures, as well as the level of humidity, uncomfortable, perhaps even unbearable. Higher temperatures can pose a cardiovascular risk by elevating heart rate and blood pressure. This concern is reduced with a FIR sauna. It is possible to burn 600 calories in 30 minutes (usually the maximum time recommended for a FIR sauna) and experience both weight loss and detoxification benefits. However, the fluid loss must be replaced with pure water (at least two cups per sauna session, in addition to at least eight to ten cups throughout the day) and minerals to prevent dehydration.

Numerous studies, the bulk of which have been published by Japanese and Chinese researchers, have made claims regarding the diverse healing benefits of FIR saunas with regard to injuries. These studies have suggested improvements in numerous ailments including arthritis, bursitis, compression fractures, muscle tension, whiplash, sciatica, soft tissue injuries and numerous other injuries, illnesses and disorders. Western studies have focused more on the sauna's ability to promote weight loss, cardiovascular conditioning and detoxification. As early as 1981, the *Journal of the American Medical Association* reported that medical research had confirmed that far-infrared saunas provide cardiovascular conditioning. This occurs as the body attempts to cool itself by increasing heart rate, cardiac output and metabolic rate.

According to J. F. Lehmann, editor of *Therapeutic Heat and Cold* (4th Edition), FIR or radiant heat therapy has been shown to:

- Increase the extensibility of collagen tissues, which means that the tissue actually extends and covers greater space. This is valuable for ligaments, tendons, fascia and other tissues that have been scarred or damaged.
- Decrease joint stiffness directly. A 20 percent decrease in stiffness in rheumatoid finger joints occurred when the ambient temperature was raised from 91°C to 113°F.
- Relieve muscle spasms. Heat has long been used to reduce muscle spasms. The peak effect is achieved with radiant heat in the far-infrared range.
- Provide pain relief. Certainly the preceding benefits would suggest a reduction in pain. Additionally, heat has been demonstrated to reduce pain by acting directly on free nerve endings in tissues and on peripheral nerves.
- Increase blood flow. When muscles are heated during a FIR sauna session, there is an increase in blood flow similar to the increase that occurs during exercise.
- Assist with inflammation. Increased peripheral circulation lessens fluid build-up in the tissues, which can reduce or eliminate inflammation and promote healing.

FIR saunas often take the shape of small "cabins" constructed of oak, cedar or other types of wood. They vary in size, with capacities ranging from one-person to six-people. There is no steam-generating device (such as hot rocks and water). FIR saunas rely on dry heat generated from ceramic heaters safely located behind vented grills throughout the unit. These saunas require a reliable electrical power source to operate but use significantly less electricity than conventional saunas. Be aware that the amount of electricity required to operate FIR saunas, and therefore the cost to operate them, can vary as much as four hundred percent.

While these units can be expensive to purchase, ranging from $3,000 to more than $5,000.00 U.S. for the larger sizes, the benefits of a daily FIR sauna may far outweigh the initial cost. Alternatively, some spas, health clubs and healing centers offer access to FIR saunas as part of their therapies and services to clients. The price ranges from $35 to $60 U.S. per half-hour session.

See the Resources for more information.

Feldenkrais Therapy

Moshe Feldenkrais, an engineer and applied physicist as well as the founder of Feldenkrais Therapy, was plagued by an old knee injury that he believed continued because of a poor pattern of movement. He studied movement of the body and specifically how to achieve body movement that would involve minimum effort and maximum efficiency.

This therapy consists of the following two separate elements: 1) functional integration and 2) awareness through movement. Functional integration involves a therapeutic session in which the practitioner uses manipulation techniques to retrain the body and mind into using more efficient movement. Awareness through movement is taught in workshops where people perform gentle exercises with the goal of bringing maximum consciousness to each activity.

Feldenkrais therapy is valuable for anyone healing from an injury, regardless of its nature, but especially spinal disorders and muscular injuries, arthritis and injuries involving chronic pain.

Herbalism or Herbal Therapy

Since human beings have been eating, we have been using herbalism to achieve healing. People in various cultures worldwide, including in China, Egypt, India, and the Americas, have accumulated knowledge of plants and their medicinal properties. This knowledge has been passed down for thousands of years to embody our modern form of herbal medicine.

Backed by thousands of past research studies (and more continually in progress), herbal medicine is a proven holistic health discipline that can provide great results with healing from injuries.

Herbalism involves the use of extracts from the leaves, seeds, bark, berries, flowers, roots, sap, or other parts of a plant. These extracts are used therapeutically as teas, tinctures, creams, poultices, elixirs, plasters, juices, syrups, decoctions and in other forms, depending on the particular herb and the medicinal use desired.

While self-administering herbs is possible, it is preferable to consult an herbalist who is trained in this powerful therapy. Under the guidance of a knowledgeable herbalist possible negative effects or drug interactions are greatly limited. Keep in mind that many other holistic health therapists use herbal medicine with their clients, but have a more limited scope in their training than herbalists.

Herbalists will take stock of your current health picture, determine what nutritional supplements and medications you are taking, and develop an herbal program accordingly. It may entail ingesting herbal teas or capsules, applying herbal creams or salves, or another approach altogether.

I urge you to consider this wonderful approach to healing your injuries and not to let the media's misinformation about particular herbs cloud your judgment. Often, when there were negative effects of herbs cited in studies, they were not properly administered or they were taken alongside a drug that interacted negatively with the herb. In these situations, typically, no one faults the synthetic, chemical drug used.

Homeopathy

Hippocrates, the father of medicine, may have been the first homeopath to discover that "like cures like," which is the basic healing principle of this discipline. However, it is Dr. Samuel Hahnemann, a German physician, who is credited with the founding of homeopathy when he experimented with diluting substances to the point that none of the original material was present, except its energetic signature. Hahnemann was motivated in his research by the harsh medical practices of his time. Working on a translation of the book *Materia Medica* by W. Cullen, he observed that the reactions of a healthy body to the use of quinine were the same as the symptoms it was used to alleviate. From this inspiration sprung his theory, "simila, simillibus curantur," or "like is healed by like," which he published in book form in 1796.

Hahnemann experimented for many years on himself and friends and family, having tremendous success with the principles he developed. The foundation of his practice is the belief that instead of using drugs that oppose and suppress the symptoms of an illness, one should use in DILUTED form a drug or medical substance that undiluted would cause that same illness. Thus, homeopathy began in full force. The word "homeopathy" is derived from two Greek words: homos, meaning "like" and pathos, meaning "suffering."

This theory may sound far-fetched to some people. However, this is the same concept on which present day medical vaccinations are based. The difference is that homeopathic remedies do not contain the harmful chemical additives and heavy metals often found in vaccines.

In homeopathy, the higher the number of the remedy, for example, 6x or 30x, the stronger it is. This number represents the degree of dilution of the active substance.

Because homeopathy is truly a holistic healing modality, a skilled practitioner will select remedies for their physical, emotional, mental and spiritual effects. So, do not be surprised if, when you consult a homeopath, he or she asks you many detailed questions. The homeopath is simply trying to get a clear picture of what your symptoms are and what worsens or improves them to select the best remedy that will produce the most effective results.

Due to its incredibly complex nature homeopathy is most effective when you use it under the guidance of a skilled practitioner, rather than trying to self-treat. Having said that, I have still included some of the main remedies that tend to be effective for common types of injuries.

A session with a homeopath will typically involve completing a detailed questionnaire, answering more questions, and a remedy or remedies prescribed to be taken for a few days, weeks or months, depending on the nature of the ailment. There is typically a follow-up appointment to assess the progress.

Lymphatic Drainage

This gentle form of massage stimulates the flow of the lymphatic system (a network of nodes covering the body that help the body eliminate toxins) and is particularly helpful for people whose injuries have created edema (swelling) although it is beneficial to everyone since most people have stagnant lymph.

Movements in this form of massage are deep, rhythmic and methodical and stretch the tissues in the direction that lymph normally flows. Some massage therapists offer "lymphatic drainage" or "lymph massage" as part of their services. The lymphatic system is intricately linked to the immune system so its stimulation is helpful for the healing of injuries. If the body is overloaded with toxins, the areas where lymph resides will tend to be sore to the touch.

Massage

There are many types of massage, ranging from "hot stone" to Swedish to Hawaiian. Massage, when administered by a trained massage therapist, can help with the healing of an injury. It is important to be aware that there are many untrained or only moderately-trained massage therapists who might be capable of handling basic massage techniques, but are not adequately skilled to deal with injuries, particularly head or spinal injuries. Always choose a massage therapist who has the training and experience necessary to handle these types of injuries.

Usually, a session entails gathering details about your medical history, including any injuries you may have had. While clothing is usually removed, a cloth will be draped over your body for warmth and to preserve modesty. Any part of the body that is not being massaged will usually remain covered.

There are forms of massage that deal exclusively with the physical body, while others work on releasing emotions, or on a more spiritual level. Choose a practitioner whose massage style suits your needs. Sessions can last for a half-hour to two hours.

Naturopathy

Naturopathy is really a collection of natural therapies such as herbalism, acupuncture, massage, homeopathy, and others. Naturopaths, the doctors who practice naturopathy, focus on nutritional counseling, natural remedies, detoxifying the body, and using holistic therapies to help the body rebuild.

A session varies greatly from one naturopath to another depending on his or her area of expertise.

Nutritional Therapy

Nutritional therapy isn't the same as dietetics, which is practiced by dieticians. Nutritional therapy is practiced by holistic nutritionists for the purpose of healing the body and employing the curative and medicinal properties in food. Dietetics tends to focus on so-called "healthy eating," which may or may not be tailored for people who want to lose weight, or have conditions like diabetes rendering them unable to eat many foods. There are some dieticians who practice holistic nutrition and nutritional therapy, but most do not.

While a holistic nutritionist may develop programs to help a person lose weight or adapt to conditions like diabetes, his or her approach is to try to help a person REGAIN HEALTH, not just LIVE WITH DISEASE.

There are many approaches to nutritional therapy. Understanding the nature of food helps us make better choices for our healing. Contrary to common belief, healthy, therapeutic food can still taste fabulous.

Nutritional therapy is as old as humans. As long as we have existed on the planet, we have been eating. Archaeological evidence suggests that ancient people ate healthier diets than we do in modern times. There is probably no more important therapy than nutritional therapy. The average person eats at least three times per day plus snacks. Many health problems can be prevented or eliminated by simply making better food choices. Because everyone is unique, the best choices may differ from person to person. There are countless reports of people who have healed from all sorts of injuries and ailments using food as the primary healing approach. It makes sense when you consider that every single cell in the human body is made up of the building blocks obtained from food. Eat poorly and you will suffer. Eat well and you will thrive.

Finding a skilled holistic nutritionist may take some effort. There are few regulations in the field of nutrition. Many of the most skilled nutritionists have learned their art over many years but I believe that in addition to hands-on experience nutritionists should also have some formal education. While there are many nutritional consultants working in health food stores who are quite knowledgeable, it has been my experience that there are many more "nutritionists" who offer dangerous and ignorant advice.

Typically a nutritionist will ask you to fill in a detailed questionnaire about your health and symptoms of illness. Some will ask you to have food sensitivity tests or laboratory nutritional tests done. He or she will then develop a dietary program to suit your particular needs. It is my experience that many people come to me claiming they already eat healthily and after some routine tests I find countless problems with their diet and vitamin, mineral or other nutritional deficiencies. You will likely achieve the best results if you have an open mind. Try the nutritional program I include in this book as part of the Eight-Week Injury- Healing Program and stick with it for at least a couple of months (with minimal cheating). The best results occur with the greatest commitment.

Osteopathy

Back in the 19th century, American doctor and engineer Andrew Taylor Still became dissatisfied with orthodox medicine and thought there must be a better approach to health. Because of his engineering background he had a unique view of the human body. He theorized that the body should run like a finely tuned engine and that much illness is directly attributable to misalignment of the body. Based on this theory, he devised a system to bring the body back into balance and return a full range of motion to the body's bones, joints, muscles and ligaments.

Thus, osteopathy was founded in 1874, and quickly became widely accepted. Dr. Still recognized that the injuries, accidents, habitually bad posture, disease, abuse or misuse of the body, or repetitive strain could lead to problems in the musculoskeletal system, thereby resulting in imbalances elsewhere in the body.

Osteopathy is an effective therapy for all of the health concerns I just mentioned, as well as many others. An osteopathic session typically begins with a detailed questionnaire of a person's medical history, followed by a thorough physical examination in a variety of normal movements and positions such as lying down, sitting, standing, and bending. This involves the osteopath applying pressure to various areas of the body to determine whether they are stressed, tense, or tired.

Each session lasts between a half-hour to an hour and is typically a very relaxing experience. Osteopaths generally employ a wide variety of techniques to help realign the body, including soft tissue manipulation, massage, and gentle movement of certain joints. Most people experience benefits after a single session. However, with acute or long-term conditions treatments may continue for months.

Osteopathy is a proven effective treatment for arthritis, asthma, back pain or injuries, bronchitis, bursitis, carpal tunnel syndrome, constipation, earaches, headaches, flu, endometriosis, hearing problems, heartburn, hemorrhoids, menstrual problems, muscle cramps, pain (acute or chronic), prostate problems, sinusitis, sports or traumatic injuries, and varicose veins.

Quantum Biofeedback

Based on more than 20 years of research in the field of bioenergetic medicine, quantum biofeedback detects, assesses, and normalizes energy imbalances in the body. Using a machine that reads the electrical response of over 8,000 factors, such as hormones, nutrient deficiencies, allergies, vertebrae, joints, parasites, emotions, and many others, the results are fed back to a computer for analysis and to administer therapies.

The system basically searches for stress patterns in the body and then administers appropriate therapies to help the body correct any imbalances found. During the sessions, a biofeedback therapist places small bands around your ankles, wrists and forehead to read the electrical and energetic responses of your body. The process is painless and usually involves sitting or lying in a comfortable chair or on a padded table. By correcting the imbalances, many people feel increased levels of energy, enhanced mental clarity, and improved healing of many types of disorders. Sessions vary in length from a half-hour to two hours depending on the nature of the health concerns, whether it is a first visit or a repeat therapy, and based on the practitioner's preference.

Reiki

Reiki (pronounced "ray-kee") is Japanese for "universal life energy." This ancient, hands-on healing art was re-discovered by Mikao Usui, a Japanese minister working at a Christian seminary in the nineteenth century. He spent many years searching for the ability to heal. After studying Buddhism and Chinese and Sanskrit to enable him to read ancient texts, Dr. Usui ventured to a sacred mountain site and fasted for 21 days, hoping to receive insight into healing.

On the twenty-first day, Usui was struck by a powerful light and saw visions of symbols that revealed to him the workings of the universal life force energy, as it was described in ancient Sanskrit writing. This gave him insight into using this universal energy to conduct healing. His insights proved accurate when he placed his hands on people and generated powerful healings.

Usui shared his knowledge and healing attunements with 16 disciples. They, in turn, helped spread this healing art to thousands of people throughout the world.

Reiki practitioners share the belief that when energy flow is restored in the body, so is health. This hands-on healing modality has undergone rigorous scientific testing and has shown proven results. Scientists suspect several factors are the basis of its success, including that the hands emit magnetic energy, an electrical charge, and infrared light that is in a healing range.

Richard Gerber, M.D., author of *Vibrational Medicine for the 21st Century*, cites a study conducted by Dr. Bernard Grad, a gerontologist at McGill University in Montreal, Canada, who developed one of the earliest tests of hands-on healing. He wanted to determine whether this form of healing was linked to the placebo effect so he designed a study that would remove the possibility of merely psychological therapeutic results. Using two sets of barley seeds, both treated with a saline solution to stunt their growth, he asked a healer to employ healing touch to only one set of the seeds. Grad was the only person to know which seeds had been exposed to healing touch to prevent the possibility of skewed results due to expectation of the touch healers. This approach addressed the phenomenon in research circles that the expectations of an outcome can actually affect the outcome. The results were astounding. After several weeks, Grad found that the seeds that had received hands-on healing had resulted in plants that sprouted more frequently, produced taller, leafier plants that produced higher levels of chlorophyll, at statistically significant levels.

Gerber cites numerous other studies using sick or injured patients that have proven the effectiveness of hands-on healing to reduce anxiety, produce deep states of relaxation (where the body achieves the greatest healing), and accelerate the healing of wounds.

Reiki sessions vary from one person to another but usually entail the Reiki Master placing his or her hands on various areas of the body while the client is fully clothed. Each session typically lasts between a half-hour to an hour.

Shiatsu

A unique blend of acupuncture with massage, shiatsu is an effective healing modality based on the principles of acupuncture but uses massage instead of needles to achieve changes in the energy meridians. "Shiatsu" is Japanese for "finger pressure." The techniques aim to reduce muscle tension, release toxins from the joints, relieve stiffness, and improve the body's energy flow.

Sessions vary in length from one shiatsu practitioner to another. The client is typically fully clothed for the session.

Thai Massage

Also known as "Thai yoga massage," this vigorous massage involves quite a workout for the client who will be guided into various yoga positions to disperse energy blockages, loosen tight muscles, and relax.

Thai massage works on energy meridians in the body and uses a lengthy series of stretches to help balance the whole body. The massage therapist applies pressure to the body using his or her fingers, thumbs, palms, elbows, knees, and feet.

This form of massage is excellent. However, it may be too vigorous for some injuries, particularly close to their onset. Later, as the injuries are further along in the healing process, it can help promote greater mobility and strength.

A session typically lasts about one to two hours and is performed on a mat on the floor while a client wears light, loose clothing. People usually feel invigorated after experiencing this massage/workout.

Which Natural Therapy Is Best?

The best healing results occur when one or more modalities of healing are added to a sound nutrition and exercise program. There are countless holistic methods that have their own unique strengths and weaknesses. My advice is to choose the ones that have the greatest appeal for you. Keep in mind, however, that the experience of a particular modality may vary greatly from one practitioner to another, so if you're not pleased with the results, consider trying a different therapist.

Therapeutic Devices

I highly recommend adding a few products to your home to assist with your healing. These include an organic mattress set, a supportive and natural pillow, a cherry pit heating/cooling pad, and a far-infrared sauna. Please see the Resources section at the end of the book to find out where to obtain these products.

Organic Cotton, Wool or Natural Latex Mattresses, Futons, Pillows and Comforters

Since many people react to the chemicals used in the production of their mattress (many of which incidentally irritate joints and soft tissues of the body and off-gas for years), I am including information about natural alternatives. I think it is tremendously important to sleep on a mattress that not only provides proper support for the spine but also does not irritate the body as it heals from injuries.

I have discovered an innovative Canadian company named Obasan that produces organic mattress sets, mattress covers, pillows, and comforters. It also manufactures an organic cherry pit pillow (either a pad or a cervical pillow) that can be heated or cooled and used for injured areas of the body.

I noticed a major improvement in my injuries after I switched to an Obasan natural latex mattress. Much of my husband's morning back pain and stiffness also subsided after we made the switch.

Obasan creates different mattresses, including: 100 percent organic cotton and pure wool, and 100 percent natural latex and pure wool. They also offer a natural box spring and slat that is made without the use of treated wood, petrochemical-based oils, and other harmful substances. In addition, the company also sells 100 percent organic cotton and wool futon mattresses, and 100 percent organic cotton mattress covers and options for their comforters.

Obasan also manufactures numerous different pillows including: the natural latex pillow, which offers a contoured design for spinal and head support and the 100 percent organic buckwheat pillow, which molds to your body.

Kapok Pillows

Another excellent pillow is the Ceiba (say-ba) pillow, an all-natural hypoallergenic bed pillow that is filled with silky yet durable fibers that have been hand-harvested from the kapok tree in the Philippines.

The kapok tree is the oldest and tallest tree in the rain forest, growing more than 200 feet high with widely spreading branches. All the leaves are shed during the dry season when it is cultivated for kapok, a light and fluffy floss fiber from the seedpod of the tree that is resistant to water and decay. After the ripe pods are harvested by hand, the seeds are removed and the fluffy fiber is meticulously cleaned and dried. After harvesting, the pod covers are composted to become organic fertilizer.

The Ceiba pillow is encased in 280-count thread cotton. It breathes because it is a natural product, and it does not circulate water well because of the fiber design. As a result, the pillow is more resistant to mould and bacteria. The pillow is easily cleaned in the washer and dryer, which fluffs it back to its original shape and inhibits the growth of allergens. While kapok is soft to the touch like down, it provides support in a way that not even synthetic materials can match. The pillow is also a natural choice for someone who suffers from allergies caused by other pillow materials such as down, feathers and synthetics.

The Ceiba pillow is produced almost entirely in the Philippines and its production does not involve cruelty to animals. The natural fiber is harvested in an environmentally responsible, sustainable manner, which respects the ecosystem and provides income to indigenous farmers, says company director Corie Laraya-Coutts. "The harvesting of the kapok pods helps maintain this vanishing ecosystem and every kapok tree left standing is a step towards the preservation of the rainforest."

Organic Cherry Pit Heating/Cooling Pad

This therapeutic heating/cooling pad is made from organic cotton stuffed with organic cherry pits. It comes in two sizes: a cervical pillow for the neck and a pad to be used on the body. It can be heated in a microwave or cooled in the freezer. It retains heat and cold longer than synthetic types of heating/cooling pads. Not only that, the cherry pits feel incredibly comfortable and offer gentle acupressure.

The manufacturer, Obasan, drop-ships to most places in the world, usually within two to three weeks.

9
FOOD PREPARATION WITH HEALING IN MIND

E ating for healing is easier and tastier than you might think. A healing regime includes a lot of fruits and vegetables prepared in gourmet dishes that help your body heal but also taste fabulous. Some of these recipes are among my favorites so do not let their healthy nature put you off. You will discover some real treasures among them and I am sure some of these recipes are sure to become your favorites as well.

Make your main dish a large, raw salad. Eat cooked food as a complement. It is actually quite simple once you make this eating pattern habitual.

Dips and Dressings

We need plenty of essential fatty acids for healing. Most people eat harmful fats and those who eat healthy ones often eat them in an inappropriate ratio. We need Omega-3 and Omega-6 fatty acids for health but most people eat 20 times the amount of Omega-6 fatty acids than Omega-3s. The problem with this disparity is that while your body requires Omega 6s, too many of them worsen pain and inflammation. Omega-3s help keep Omega-6s in check. The salad dressing that follows is very high in Omega-3 fatty acids.

In addition, one of the best foods for arthritic types of pains is apple cider vinegar, which I have used in this recipe to maximize its pain-fighting properties. Be sure to use apple cider vinegar that contains live culture, known as the "mother." Blueberries are excellent pain-fighters as well. They contain a substance that is ten times more potent than aspirin at fighting pain and inflammation.

Pain-Reducing Salad Dressing .

> 1/2 cup blueberries (fresh or frozen)
> 3/4 cup cold-pressed refrigerated flax-seed oil
> 1/3 cup apple cider vinegar (with sediment in the bottom, purchased at a health food store)
> a dash of Celtic sea salt
> 1 tbsp pure maple syrup

Blend with a hand mixer or whisk together. If whisking ingredients together, mash the blueberries with a fork. Pour over mixed baby greens since they have the greatest healing properties of various types of lettuce.

Inflammation-Beating Salad Dressing

> 3/4 cup cold-pressed refrigerated flax-seed oil
> 1/3 cup apple cider vinegar (with sediment in the bottom and purchased at a health food store)
> 1/2 tsp Celtic sea salt
> 1/2 tsp basil
> 1/2 tsp thyme
> 1/2 tsp oregano
> a dash of cayenne pepper

Bone-Building Salad Dressing/Dip

> 1/2 cup raw tahini (mashed sesame seeds found in most health food stores or Lebanese or Middle Eastern markets)
> 2 lemons (Do NOT substitute Realemon or other lemon products. These products have been cooked, making them acidic in the body. Fresh lemon is alkalizing to the body, which is essential to allow your body to absorb the large amount of calcium in this dressing.)
> 1 clove fresh garlic
> 1-2 tbsp cold-pressed flax oil
> pure water (as needed to obtain the desired consistency)

Blend all the ingredients together, adding water until you obtain the desired consistency. Use more water for a salad dressing, less for a vegetable dip. This dressing can be used in place of Caesar salad dressing or as a delicious dip for crudités. It is packed with a huge amount of calcium.

Guacamole

This recipe makes an excellent veggie dip or sandwich spread. Use soon after making it or it will discolor.

    1 avocado, pitted and peeled
    1 small clove garlic
    1/2 lime
    a dash of Celtic sea salt
    1 tbsp cold-pressed flax oil

Blend all ingredients together until creamy, using a hand mixer or food processor. Serve with vegetable crudités, such as carrot, celery, red or green pepper sticks, broccoli or cauliflower.

Juices, Smoothies and Teas

Anti-Inflammatory Juice

    6 large carrots (remove tops)
    1 apple
    1-inch piece of ginger

Pass all ingredients through a juicer. Drink immediately.

Pain-Busting Juice

    1/2 pineapple, outer skin removed (juice the core as well
        as the flesh)
    1-inch piece of ginger

Pass all ingredients through a juicer. Dilute with pure water to taste. Drink immediately.

Blood-Cleansing Juice

Dandelion is useful for cleansing the blood, which removes toxins from the tissues and joints, thereby speeding healing and lessening pain and inflammation. Be aware that if you drink a fair amount of this juice over a short period of time it can speed up the cleansing reaction, which initially might produce symptoms like fatigue or headaches. These will pass as your body becomes "cleaner."

    3 apples
    a handful of fresh dandelion (if you're digging it yourself,
        be sure to obtain organic dandelion where the land hasn't

been sprayed for several years and is far removed from
traffic areas)
Pass all ingredients through a juicer. Drink immediately.

Pain-Away Pina Colada

2-inch thick slice of fresh pineapple, core and outer skin
removed
1 can coconut milk (this is one of the only canned foods
included in my Healing Food Pyramid)
Blend in a blender with 8–10 ice cubes. Serve immediately.

Cranberry Anti-Pain Cocktail

This juice when drunk regularly helps eliminate inflammation because of
the high amount of Vitamin C found in cranberries.
3 apples
1 cup cranberries
Pass all ingredients through a juicer. Dilute with water. If you are
using frozen cranberries, juice only the apples, add pure water and blend
the juice together with the cranberries in a blender. Drink immediately.

Pain Elimination Tea

Purchase dried herbs at your local health food store.
1/2 cup black aldertree
3/4 cup white willow bark
1/4 cup red sandalwood
1 cup bittersweet
1/2 cup juniper berries
1/2 cup senna
3/4 cup elder
1/2 cup primrose flowers
1 tbsp common ladies mantle
Mix all dried ingredients into a jar for future use. Shake to blend
together well. Use 1 teaspoon of dried herb in a tea strainer. Infuse for
three to five minutes. Drink three cups per day. The jar of bulk herbs
should last at least two to three months.

Celery Anti-Inflammatory Juice

1 cucumber
4 stalks celery
1–2 apples (depending on preferred sweetness)

Pass all ingredients through a juicer. Drink immediately.

Tropical Enzyme Blast

1/2 papaya (seeded and peeled)
1 mango (pitted and peeled)
1 frozen banana
1-inch slice of fresh pineapple (cored and outer skin removed)
1–2 cups water (depending on desired consistency)
Blend all ingredients in a blender or food processor. Drink immediately.

Blue Raspberry Anti-Inflammatory Smoothie

1 cup raspberries (fresh or frozen)
1 cup blueberries (fresh or frozen)
1 banana (frozen)
11/2–2 cups water (depending on desired consistency)
Blend all ingredients together. Drink immediately.

Cranberry Melon Power Juice

2 large slices watermelon
1/2 cup blueberries
1/2 cup cranberries
Push all ingredients through a juicer. Serve over ice if desired.

Almond Milk

1/4 cup raw, unsalted almonds
1 cup water
1/2 tsp unpasteurized honey or 2 drops of liquid stevia (found in most health food stores)
Blend all ingredients together until smooth. Strain if desired. Drink on its own or use as a base for smoothies.

Salads

Make salads the focal point of your meals. That might sound boring but there really are a tremendous number of delectable salads you can make if you vary the ingredients. Here is a list to help you get started. Use your creativity.

- mixed greens (mesclun)
- romaine lettuce
- Boston lettuce
- leaf lettuce
- radicchio
- pea shoots
- alfalfa sprouts
- broccoli sprouts
- onion sprouts
- clover sprouts
- mung bean sprouts
- chickpeas
- kidney beans
- pinto beans
- lima beans
- Great Northern beans
- any other type of legume
- sliced strawberries
- apple slices
- orange slices
- grapefruit slices
- avocado
- green peppers
- red peppers
- yellow peppers
- finely-chopped broccoli
- cucumber
- olives
- edible flowers
- grated carrots
- fresh peas
- grated cabbage
- chopped parsley
- chopped cilantro
- mushrooms (raw or cooked)
- green onion
- raspberries
- blueberries
- celery

Healing 5-Bean Salad

    1 can cooked and rinsed mixed beans (such as kidney, garbanzo, pinto, etc.)

    2 stalks finely chopped celery

    1 finely chopped purple onion

    1 finely chopped green pepper

    1 finely chopped red pepper

    1 finely chopped green onion

    a handful of chopped raw green or yellow beans

    3/4 cup cold-pressed, refrigerated flax-seed oil

    1/3 cup apple cider vinegar (with sediment in the bottom and purchased at a health food store)

    1/2 tsp Celtic sea salt

    1 tbsp pure maple syrup

    1/2 tsp basil

    1/2 tsp thyme

    1/2 tsp oregano

    a dash of cayenne pepper

Mix the cooked beans and chopped vegetables together in a bowl. In a jar whisk together the flax-seed oil, apple cider vinegar, Celtic sea salt, maple syrup, basil, thyme oregano and cayenne pepper. Pour half of the dressing over the bean and vegetable mixture. For the best taste, let marinate overnight or a couple of hours. Store the remaining dressing in a covered jar in the refrigerator for later use.

Mexican Salad

    one head of leaf or romaine lettuce, washed and dried

    1 tomato, chopped into cubes

    1 avocado, chopped into cubes

    1 lime

    1 small clove garlic

    a dash of Celtic sea salt

    a handful of fresh cilantro (coriander)

    1 tbsp cold-pressed flax oil

Cut or tear the lettuce and place in bowls to form a base for the other salad ingredients. Place tomato, avocado, Celtic sea salt, cilantro and flax oil together in a separate bowl. Squeeze the juice of the lime over the other ingredients. Chop or press garlic into the bowl with the other ingredients. Toss ingredients together. Serve tomato/avocado mixture over the salad greens.

Complementary Dishes

Millet

> 1 cup whole millet
> 21/2 cups water
> a dash of olive oil
> a dash of Celtic sea salt

Put all ingredients into a pot. Cover and bring to a boil. Reduce heat and let simmer on low for 45 minutes. Serve on its own or as a base for steamed or stir-fried vegetables.

Mexican Bruschetta

> 4 toasted slices of 100 percent whole grain bread, such as rye, spelt, or kamut
> 1 tomato, chopped into cubes
> 1 avocado, chopped into cubes
> 1/2 lime
> 1 small clove garlic, pressed or chopped finely
> a dash of Celtic sea salt
> a handful of fresh cilantro (coriander)
> 1 tbsp cold-pressed flax oil

While the bread is toasting, mix all the other ingredients into a bowl (except the lime). Squeeze the limejuice over the other ingredients. Toss together. Spoon the tomato/avocado mixture over the bread and serve.

Veggie Wrap

> 1–2 carrots, shredded
> 1/2 cucumber, sliced
> 1/2 red and/or green pepper, sliced into strips
> 1–2 tomatoes, sliced
> Or, use other raw vegetables, sliced, chopped, or grated
> 2–4 soft, preservative-free tortilla shells
> guacamole (see preceding recipe)

Spread guacamole in the center of the tortilla shells. Place a handful of each raw vegetable in a line in the center of the tortilla and roll into a wrap.

Lentil Dahl

Lentil Dahl is a delicious curried lentil dish. I modified the traditional recipe slightly to give it even greater injury-healing properties. Even if you are not a huge fan of lentils, give this healing recipe a try.

    1 yam, cubed
    2 tbsp extra-virgin olive oil
    1 large onion, chopped
    1/2 teaspoon mustard seeds
    4 dried red chilies
    1-inch piece of ginger, grated
    2 cloves garlic, chopped
    1/2 tsp turmeric
    1 tsp Celtic sea salt
    3 cups cooked lentils, or two small cans (rinsed)
    fresh cilantro (coriander), if desired

In a medium to large pot, boil the cubed yams in water until soft. Pour off any excess water, leaving enough to mash the yams with a hand blender to a smooth consistency. In a frying pan, cook the onion, mustard seeds, chilies, ginger, and garlic in the olive oil over low heat until the onion is transparent. Add the onion mixture to the mashed yams. Then, add the lentils, turmeric, Celtic sea salt and 1/2 cup water. Stir together. Let simmer over low heat until warmed and the flavors mingle. Serve in bowls with fresh cilantro as a garnish.

Desserts

Yes, your eyes are not deceiving you. Desserts. Read on.

Cashew Cream

    1 cup raw, unsalted cashews
    1/2–1 cup water, depending on the desired cream consis-
        tency
    2 tsp unpasteurized honey

Blend all ingredients together until creamy. Serve with fresh blueberries, strawberries or other fruit.

Berry Blast Ice Cream
> 1 cup frozen raspberries
> 1 cup frozen blueberries
> 2 frozen bananas
> Blend all ingredients in a food processor.

Anti-Pain Remedy

Mix 1/2 cup of organic turmeric (spice available from most health food stores) with 1/2 cup of raw, unpasteurized honey. Store in a sealed jar and consume one to four teaspoons daily.

10
EIGHT-WEEK INJURY-HEALING PROGRAM

The Eight-Week Injury-Healing Program is a powerful tool to assist your body with healing and ensure a speedy and full recovery. Eight weeks is a sufficient amount of time to heal most injuries However, in the case of more serious injuries, old injuries that never healed properly, or injuries that are the result of long-term depletion of the body (such as fractures from osteoporosis) I suggest that you continue with this healing program beyond the eight weeks until you are totally satisfied with the results. In all truth, you may decide to extend the program because you are feeling so great as a result of it.

To optimize your healing, you must make a commitment to follow on a daily basis all five components of the program. The five components are:

1. Eating healthily;
2. Using nutritional, herbal and/or homeopathic remedies;
3. Doing breathing and physical exercises;
4. Incorporating appropriate adjunct therapies; and
5. Maintaining a positive attitude.

Component 1: Healthy Eating

Eating well is critical to your success on this program. Since foods and water create the building blocks of every cell in your body, it is essential that you provide your body with the best possible raw materials. In this way, you will ensure superior results. It is also imperative that you avoid foods that can damage cells or waste their energy to eliminate toxins.

So, your first step during the next eight weeks (or more if you choose to extend the program) is to refrain from eating "foods," which in my opinion are more aptly termed "toxins masquerading as foods."

Foods to Avoid While Recovering from Injuries

- All processed, packaged, or fast foods (they aggravate pain, inflammation and injuries);
- All hydrogenated fats (margarine, shortening, lard or products made with them such as cookies, pies, packaged foods, buns, etc.);
- All meat (steaks, burgers, lamb, chicken, turkey, duck, Cornish hen, etc.);
- All fried foods (French fries, onion rings, potato chips, nachos, hamburgers, etc., since they contribute to toxicity, acidity, and increase pain and inflammation);
- All white sugar (and foods made from this sweet);
- All other sugars (brown sugar, cane sugar, turbinado sugar, demarrara sugar, molasses, beet sugar, date sugar—although a small amount of honey is permitted as is stevia, a herb that is naturally one thousand times sweeter than sugar);
- All synthetic sweeteners (Nutrasweet, saccharin, aspartame, etc.);
- Salt (use Celtic sea salt instead);
- All food additives (colors, flavor enhancers, stabilizers, preservatives, etc.);
- All white flour products (breads, pastries, pasta, etc.);
- All dairy products (yogurt, ice cream, cottage cheese, butter, cheese, etc.);
- All wheat products (wheat, even whole wheat is very acidifying and can counter the benefits of the program);
- Coffee and black tea (green tea and herbal teas are permitted);
- All soft drinks, sweetened juices, fruit punch and other sweetened beverages; and
- All alcohol.

I also suggest that you limit your sodium intake and use instead Celtic sea salt.

Foods to Eat While Recovering from Injuries

- Plenty of raw fruits and berries, such as apples, pineapple, cherries, blueberries, blackberries, raspberries and strawberries;

- Plenty of raw vegetables, such as celery, tomatoes and bell peppers and leafy greens, such as spinach, dandelion greens and kale;
- Plenty of cooked vegetables;
- Fatty fish such as salmon, mackerel, herring, sardines, and tuna;
- Flax oil, walnut oil, hemp oil, or extra virgin olive oil;
- Spices like turmeric, garlic, cloves, onions, ginger, celery seeds, turmeric, chili peppers, licorice (the herb, not the candy), peppermint, and paprika;
- Plenty of fresh juices made at home in a juicer from raw vegetables and fruits;
- Fresh raw and unsalted nuts, especially walnuts and almonds;
- Whole grains and legumes;
- Soy foods: soymilk, tofu (but not the heavily processed soy derivatives like hot dogs, luncheon meats, etc.);
- Stevia (to sweeten foods or beverages, if desired);
- Green tea or herbal teas; and
- Green food supplements.

A Note About Green Food Supplements

Green food supplements are any type of green powder such as spirulina, barley juice, and chlorella. Two of my favorites are Barley Max and Greens Rx. Barley Max is processed at low temperatures to retain the enzymes and nutrients. It is made from the juice of organic barley grass and alfalfa and is a powerhouse of nutrients, including vitamins, minerals, amino acids, and trace minerals. Unlike many green food products, it dissolves in water or juice, making it more palatable and easier to mix.

Greens Rx is an excellent green food supplement, which has been processed at low temperatures to ensure the greatest amount of enzymes and nutrients (this is rare with green food supplements). It is available in many health food stores. It includes: lecithin, Hawaiian spirulina, high pectin apple fiber, organic kamut juice powder, organic alfalfa powder, organic barley juice powder, organic red beet juice powder, organic brown rice germ and bran, organic soy sprouts, organic sprouted barley malt, dairy free probiotic culture, royal jelly, bee pollen, acerola berry juice powder, licorice root powder, and Pacific kelp.

Please see the Resources section at the end of the book for purchasing information.

Cellfood® is a unique cell-oxygenating liquid formula that delivers 78 trace minerals, 34 enzymes, 17 amino acids and electrolytes. It is readily absorbed by the body at the cellular level, making a wealth of nutrients available to your cells for optimum healing. According to the manufacturer, Cellfood® increases the bioavailability of oxygen to the body. Unlike most other oxygen products, Cellfood® delivers the oxygen slowly, thereby preventing free radical damage. Cellfood® also helps normalize the pH of the body. It actually helps alkalize an acidic body, which is integral to proper healing. This helps create an overall acid-alkaline balance in the blood and tissues of the body. It also assists with energy, boosts the immune system, and detoxifies the body. I recommend taking this product three times per day in a glass of pure water. It contains the following essential nutrients:

Oxygen

Trace Minerals:	actinium, antimony, argon, astatine, barium, beryllium, bismuth, boron, bromine, calcium, carbon, cerium, cesium, chromium, cobalt, copper, dysprosium, erbium, europium, fluorine, gadolinium, gallium, germanium, gold, hafnium, helium, holmium, hydrogen, indium, iodine, iridium, iron, krypton, lanthanum, lithium, lutetium, magnesium, manganese, molybdenum, neodymium, neon, nickel, niobium, nitrogen, osmium, oxygen, palladium, phosphorous, platinum, polonium, potassium, praseodymium, promethium, rhenium, rhodium, rubidium, ruthenium, samarium, selenium, silica, silicon, silver, sodium, sulfur, tantalum, technetium, tellurium, terbium, thallium, thorium, tin, titanium, tungsten, vanadium, xenon, ytterbium, zinc, and zirconium (does not contain aluminium, cadmium, chlorine, mercury, lead, or radium)

Metabolic Enzymes	hydrolases, carbohydrases: maltase, sucrase, emulsin
	nucleases: polynucleotidase, nucleotidase
	hydrases: fumarase, enolase
	peptidases: aminopolypeptidase, dipeptidase, prolinase
	copper enzymes: tyrosinase, ascorbic acid oxidase
	esterase: lipase, phosphotase, sulfatase
	iron enzymes: catalase, cytochrome oxidase, peroxidase
	enzymes containing coenzymes 1 and/or 2: lactic dehy
	drogenase, robison ester dehydrogenase
	yellow enzymes: Warburg's yellow enzymes, diaphorase, Haas enzyme, cytochrome C reductase
	enzymes that reduce cytochrome: succinic dehydrogenase
	aidase: urease
	mutases: aldehyde mutase, glyoxalase
	desmolases: zymohexase, carboxylase
	other enzymes: phosphorylase, phosphohexisomerase, hexokinase, phosphoglumutase
Amino Acids:	alanine, arginine, aspartic acid, cystine, glutamic acid, glycine, histidine, isoleucine, lysine, methionine, phenylalanine, proline, serine, threonine, tryptophan, tyrosine, valine

Electrolytes

Cellfood® is available from many health food stores or healthcare practitioners. See the Resources section at the back of this book for additional information.

Healing Food Pyramid

Once again, I urge you to use the Healing Food Pyramid and the corresponding Healing Foods Chart as both a reference and a guide. Consider photocopying both of these and posting them on your fridge as a daily reminder of the healing foods you should be eating

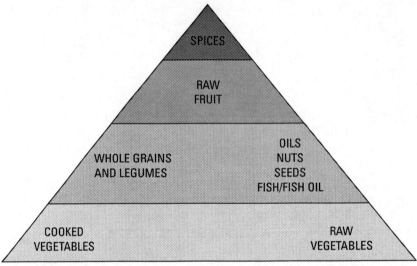

As you can see from the Healing Food Pyramid diagram, the bulk of your foods should be eaten in a raw state. There are countless ways to prepare raw fruits and vegetables and a multitude of ingredients that you can easily incorporate into salads. You will find some wonderful healing recipes in chapter 9. Most of the raw foods you eat should be vegetables and freshly pressed vegetable juices. A lesser amount of raw foods can include cold-pressed flax, olive, hemp, or walnut oil. Nuts and seeds should be eaten raw and unsalted.

To help you with your food choices, please use the Healing Foods Chart that follows which lists the best foods for each category of the Healing Food Pyramid and the top anti-inflammatory and anti-pain foods.

Healing Foods Chart*

Top Anti-Inflammatory and Anti-Pain Spices	Raw Fruit	Whole Grains** & Legumes	Oils***, Nuts****, Seeds, Fish & Fish Oils	Vegetables(Mostly Raw)	Top Anti-Inflammatory & Anti-Pain Foods	Foods with Natural Aspirin to Counter Pain	Top Calcium-Rich Body-Alkalizing Foods (in order of calcium potency)
Turmeric	Pineapple	Millet	Walnut oil	Mesclun	Cherries	Blueberries	Sesame
Celery	Papaya	Quinoa	Flax oil	(mixed	and cherry	Cherries	seeds
seeds	Mango	Brown	Hemp oil	greens)	juice	Dried	Seaweed,
Garlic	Lemon	rice	X-virgin	Romaine	Blueberries	currants	agar
Ginger	Lime	Spelt	olive oil	lettuce	Celery	Curry	Seaweed,
Cloves	Grapefruit	Kamut	Walnuts	Boston	Tomatoes	powder	dulse
Chili	Orange	Kidney	Hazelnuts	lettuce	(raw)	Dates	Collard
peppers	Kiwi	beans	Almonds	Radicchio	Bell pepper	Gherkins	leaves
(capsaicin)	Grapes	Garbanzo	Pecans	Pea shoots	(raw)	Licorice	Kale leaves
Licorice	Rhubarb	beans	Pistachios	Alfalfa	Pineapple	herb	Turnip
(herb)	Pears	Lentils	Sunflower	sprouts	Fatty fish	Paprika	greens
Peppermint	Apples	Lima beans	seeds	Broccoli	(salmon,	Prunes	Almonds**
Paprika	Avocado	Pinto beans	Pumpkin	sprouts	tuna,	Rasp-	***
Onion	Blueberries	Romano	seeds	Onion	mackerel	berries	Soy beans
	Cherries	beans	Sesame	sprouts	& herring)		Hazelnuts
	Black-		seeds	Clover	Flax oil		(filberts)
	berries		Salmon	sprouts	and walnut		Brazil
	Rasp-		Mackerel	Mung bean	oil		nuts****
	berries		Herring	sprouts	Walnuts		Parsley
	Straw-		Tuna	Avocado	Spinach		Collard
	berries			Green/red/	Kale		stems
				yellow	Dandelion		Dandelion
				peppers	Apples		greens
				Broccoli	Onion		Mustard
				Cucumber	Dried		greens
				Carrots	currants		Kale stems
				Peas	Dates		Watercress
				Cabbage	Gherkins		Pepper
				Sweet	(small		(red hot)
				potatoes	cucum		Chick peas
				Yams	bers)		Sunflower
				Fennel	Prunes		seeds
				Bok choy	(unsul		Beet
				Fiddle-	phured)		greens
				heads	Rasp-		Mung bean
				Tomatoes	berries		sprouts
				(raw)	Black-		Brocolli
				Celery	berries		Fennel

173

*   Do not assume that if a particular fruit or vegetable or berry does not appear on this list that it shouldn't be eaten or has no healing properties. I simply tried to include all the top ones in each category.

**   Avoid wheat products since they're very acidic and many people are sensitive to them. If you're celiac or have gluten sensitivity, you can still eat healthily following the remainder of the Healing Food Pyramid.

***   All oils should be cold-pressed and ideally bought in a health food store.

**** Avoid peanuts since they tend to contain many aflatoxins (mold-like substances), which aggravate joints and inflame tissues.

***** Nuts are only alkalizing if they are raw and unsalted.

A Typical Day in the Eight-Week Injury-Healing Program

Morning

Drink a glass of water with eight drops of Cellfood® in it when you first awaken. Fifteen minutes later, take your green food supplement in a small amount of unsweetened juice or water on an empty stomach. Start by taking 1/2 teaspoon twice daily for the first week. Then, increase to 1 teaspoon twice daily. Wait 15 minutes before eating breakfast. Finally, eat a breakfast consisting of any of the foods on the list of Foods to Eat on the Eight-Week Injury-Healing Program, but do include raw foods.

Mid-Morning

Take one heaping teaspoon of the turmeric-honey anti-pain mixture.

Lunch

Lunch can consist of any of the foods on the list of Foods to Eat on the Eight-Week Injury-Healing Program but should include a large, raw salad with flax oil dressing or the Bone-Building Salad Dressing (See recipes in Chapter 9).

Mid-Afternoon

Drink a glass of water with eight drops of Cellfood® in it. Fifteen minutes later, take your green food supplement in a small amount of unsweetened juice or water.

Dinner

Your dinner can consist of any of the foods on the list of Foods to Eat on the Eight-Week Injury-Healing Program, but should include a large, raw salad with flax oil dressing or the Bone-Building Salad Dressing (see recipes in Chapter 9).

Evening Snack

If desired, munch on raw fruits or vegetable sticks with a dip.

Before Bed

Drink a glass of water with eight drops of Cellfood® in it.

Throughout the Day...

In addition to this daily regimen, do not drink with meals. Wait at least one hour after meals to drink, and drink at least eight cups of pure water throughout the day.

Component 2: Nutritional, Herbal and/or Homeopathic Remedies

I have already discussed two of the powerful tools in this component that you should incorporate in your healing program—a green food supplement and Cellfood®. In addition, various herbs and homeopathic remedies can also enhance your healing process. You must select herbs and/or homeopathic remedies to suit your symptoms. Please review the information on this topic in chapters 1, 2, 3, and 5.

Component 3: Breathing and Physical Exercises

I recommend you include four types of exercise several times per week in your Eight-Week Injury-Healing Program. They are:

1. stretching (like the stretching exercises shown in chapter 6);
2. strengthening (weight or resistance training);
3. cardiovascular (any exercise that gets your heart rate up); and
4. breathing (an excellent way to center your mind and clear it from the clutter of the day as well as to bring oxygen to all the cells of your body).

Start your exercise program gradually and work your way up to longer duration, greater weight, or more repetitions.

Component 4: Adjunct Therapies

Also, if desired, use a therapy or two from the many types mentioned in chapter 8. Be sure to select a therapy that suits your personality, injury, and approach to healing.

Component 5: Maintaining a Positive Attitude

In chapter 1, I explained that there is a clear connection between stress and bone loss. In countless studies, research shows that stress or a negative outlook has an impact on many other health issues. It can greatly diminish healing ability, depress the immune system, increase damaging hormones, and decrease energy. While you may not always feel great about the injury you sustained or the way it prevents you from doing certain activities, it is important to allow yourself to have those feelings and then move on to allow your body to heal. There are many effective ways to release negative feelings, including: confiding in a partner or close friend, writing your feelings out, or crying if you need to. Recognize that you are simply feeling down for a moment in time, a moment that can just as easily be turned to create a positive outlook.

Make sure you eliminate whatever stress you can and try to find the blessing in the stress you feel powerless to change.

Also, ensure you get enough sleep. If pain is affecting your sleep, try the foods and remedies I suggested earlier. Also, warm baths can help with sleep and relaxation.

Healing Baths

Every day, soak in a warm bath with 1/2 cup of baking soda added to the water. This alkalizes the water, which in turn, helps alkalize your blood. Slightly alkaline blood enables the body to heal faster, reducing pain and inflammation. Soak for at least twenty minutes. If you have excessive inflammation you may want to wait until some of the swelling dissipates before immersing the injured area into warm water.

Before retiring to bed, dissolve about one pound of Epsom salts into a warm bath. Soak for about twenty minutes. When you are finished, do not rub yourself dry. Instead, wrap up in several warm towels and go to bed immediately. This will help your body detoxify and heal. Avoid Epsom salt baths if you are diabetic, feel tired or weak, or have heart trouble.

Tailoring the Eight-Week Injury-Healing Program to Your Injury

If you are healing from a bone injury, incorporate some of the suggested remedies in chapter 1. If you injured the soft tissues of your body, incorporate the suggestions in chapter 2. Likewise, if you sustained a joint injury, follow the suggestions made in chapter 3.

If you are suffering from pain or inflammation, increase your consumption of anti-inflammatory, anti-pain foods as mentioned in chapter 4 or add some of the natural remedies suggested in chapter 5.

Keep a daily record of the foods you eat at breakfast, lunch and dinner, along with any snacks throughout the day, whether you ate 50 percent of your foods raw and drank at least eight cups of water daily. Note any foods you ate that are not part of the program to help you keep track of items that may hinder your progress. Also, list the nutritional and herbal supplements. This may sound tedious but it will enable you to observe patterns between increases and decreases in pain or inflammation or to discover foods that might be hindering your healing.

11

MAXIMIZING YOUR INJURY HEALING

Now that you have learned some of the essential principles of healing injuries, you have probably already started putting them into practice. I certainly hope so. Much of what you have learned constitutes sound health principles that you can carry with you throughout your life, to maintain not only the health of the injured area you have healed but many other aspects of your health as well.

As you read in chapter 4, one of the greatest weapons against injury and disease is nutrition. Food really is the best medicine (not to mention the most readily attainable, cost-effective, and best-tasting). Eating a diet high in raw fruits and vegetables is a powerful way to prevent injuries from worsening, help them heal, and prevent them from returning. It is also an excellent way to help ward off some of the serious chronic diseases we face in the twenty-first century.

Continuing to make raw fruits and vegetables at least 50 percent of your food selection (by visible portions, not by calories) is a simple task. Include a large and varied salad with your lunch and dinner meals, snack on raw fruits and crudités. Make breakfast partially (or fully) raw fruits.

Become acquainted with the foods that increase inflammation and pain and those that lessen it. Choose only foods that will help your body heal and feel more comfortable. Such simple solutions to pain and inflammation really do make a difference over the long term. You will notice tremendous improvements if you stick to this way of eating. Simply follow the Healing Food Pyramid as your guide to making better food choices. If you need additional support, try the natural herbs, aromatherapy oils, or homeopathic remedies suggested in chapter 5 as well as the healing modalities discussed in chapter 8.

Of course, do not forget exercise. As your body heals, continue to make exercise a regular part of your life. Not only is it helpful in pain reduction, it can make your body less vulnerable to further injury. Plus, it will create more energy for healing. Make sure to include regular stretching exercises, like those described in chapter 6, along with cardiovascular and strength training exercise. Incorporating all three types of exercise produces the best results.

Once you complete the Eight-Week Injury-Healing Program, you may be tempted to dive into a large plate of French fries or a big steak. I urge you to reconsider. Although, if you choose to, you may witness a resurgence of pain in your body and what better motivation to continue your healthy eating habits than to experience pain once again. On the flip side, you may be feeling so great that you want to continue eating and living your life as you have on the Eight-Week Injury-Healing Program. That is great too.

I have personally experienced the rewards of sticking with this type of program and the pain of falling off the program, as have many others. Most people also observe other nagging complaints subside when they follow this way of eating and living. They may lose weight (if overweight), have more energy, feel greater mental clarity, observe skin or sinus problems clear, and experience a multitude of other health improvements. I hope this happens for you as well. After all, sound therapeutic nutrition not only helps heal injuries, it helps heal people's bodies.

Be patient, persistent, and diligent. You will be happy you were. I wish you tremendous success on your healing journey.

RESOURCES

Sleeping Aids

For information on organic cotton, wool or natural latex mattress sets, futons, pillows, comforters, and therapeutic cherry pit heating/cooling cushions:

Obasan
50 Colonnade Road, Ottawa, ON
K2E 7J6
Canada
Tel: (in Canada) 1-888-413-4442; (in the U.S) 1-800-313-3799
www.obasan.ca.

For information on Ceiba kapok pillows:

Desalon
Email: Info@desalon.com.

Nutrition Supplements

For information on Barley Max green food supplement:

Hallelujah Acres
900 S. Post Road, Shelby, NC
28152
U.S.A.
Tel: 1-800-915-well
www.hacres.com
www.barleymax.com

For information on Greens Rx supplement:

Enerex Botanicals Ltd.
8531 Eastlake Drive, Burnaby, BC
V5A 4T7
Canada
Tel: 604-422-8777
Fax: 604-422-8778
Email: info@enerex.ca
www.enerex.ca

For information on Cellfood®:
Lumina Health Products
Tel in Canada and the U.S.: 1-800-749-9196
Tel international: 941-371-3322
Fax: 941-379-2522
Email: info@luminahealth.com
www.luminahealth.com

Exercise Videos

For pilates:
Pilates Beginning Mat Workout
By Ana Caban
Produced by Living Arts
Available in many bookstores,
Or by calling 1-800-2-LIVING,
Or visiting *www.gaiam.com*

For qigong:
Qigong: Traditional Chinese Exercises for Healing Body, Mind & Spirit
By Ken Cohen
Produced and distributed by Sounds True
Available by calling 1-800-333-9185

Spring Forest Qigong for Health (Level 1)
By Chunyi Lin
Produced and distributed by Learning Strategies Corporation
Available by calling 1-800-735-8273; or 1-952-476-9200
Or visiting *www.learningstrategies.com*

Bliss Qigong, Power Qigong, Vitality Qigong, or Serenity Qigong
(four separate videos available individually)
By John Du Cane
Produced by Dragon Door Publications Inc.
Available by calling 1-800-899-5111; or 1-651-645-0517

For yoga:
Healing Yoga for Common Conditions
By Charles and Lisa Matkin
Produced by Andrea Ambandos, Dragonfly Productions Inc.
Distributed by Anchor Bay Entertainment Inc.
Available in many department stores
Or by calling 1-877-B-IN-YOGA (246-9642)
Or visiting www.livingyoga.com

Power Yoga (Stamina or Strength) for Beginners
By Rodney Yee
Produced by Living Arts
Available in many bookstores
Or by calling 1-800-2-LIVING
Or visiting www.livingarts.com

BIBLIOGRAPHY

"Avoiding Injury Spasm and Pain" (informational flyer). Advanced Nutrition Publications, Inc.:1995.

"Asian American Women and Osteoporosis." Compiled by The Florida Osteoporosis Prevention and Education Program.

Balch, M.D., James and Balch, CNC, Phyllis. *Prescription for Nutritional Healing: Second Edition.* Avery Publishing Group, New York: 1997.

Burke, Ph.D., Edmund R. *Herbs for Sports Performance, Energy and Recovery.* Keats Publishing, Inc. New Canaan, CT: 1998.

Carper, Jean. *Food—Your Miracle Medicine: Preventing and Curing Common Health Problems the Natural Way.* Harper Collins, New York: 1993.

Diamond, Harvey. *The Fit for Life Solution: How to Identify and Successfully Eradicate the Causes of Pain, Fatigue and Disease - NOW!* Dragon Door Publications, Inc., St Paul: 2002.

Forem, Jack and Shimer, LAc, Steve. *Healing with Pressure Point Therapy: Simple, Effective Techniques for Massaging Away More than 100 Common Ailments.* Prentice Hall, Paramus, NJ: 1999.

Gerber, M.D., Richard. *Vibrational Medicine for the 21st Century: The Complete Guide to Energy Healing and Spiritual Transformation.* Eagle Brook, New York: 2002.

Higley, Connie and Higley, Alan. *Aromatherapy A-Z.* Carlsbad, CA: 1998.

Jayasuriya, Anton. *Clinical Acupuncture: Seventeenth Revised and Enlarged Edition.* Chandrakanthi Press International (Pvt) Ltd., Sri Lanka: 1993.

Jensen, Bernard. *Dr. Jensen's Guide to Body Chemistry & Nutrition.* Keats Publishing, Los Angeles: 2000.

Keith, David. "Build Stronger Bones Naturally," *Health 'N Vitality Magazine.* Kirkland, Quebec, February 2002.

Lehmann, J.F. (ed.). *Therapeutic Heat and Cold, 4th Edition.* Williams & Wilkins, Baltimore, MD: 1990.

Moore, A.H.G., Martha. *Beyond Cortisone.* Keats Publishing, Los Angeles: 1999.

Morgan, Lyle W. *Homeopathic Treatment of Sports Injuries.* Healing Arts Press: 1988.

Nutri-Notes: "Integrating the Nutrition-Health Connection," Volume 1, #2, March-April 1994.

"Osteoporosis Facts: What Asian Women Need to Know." Retrieved online from the University of Washington Women's Health National Center for Excellence (*http://depts.washington.edu/uwcoe/healthtopics/ osteo/facts_asianw.html*).

Pallas, Andrew. *Beating Sports Injuries through Conventional and Alternative Methods.* Barrons Educational Series, Inc., Hauppage, NY: 2002.

Purkh Singh Shalsa, C.D.-N, R.H., Karta. "Fighting Fibromyalgia: You Can Find Natural Relief from This Complex Mystifying Disease," *Herbs for Health.* May/June 2003.

Rippe, M.D., James M. *The Joint Health Prescription: 8 Weeks to Stronger, Healthier, Younger Joints.* Rodale Inc.: 2001.

Simester, Lisha. *The Natural Health Bible.* Whitecap Books, North Vancouver: 2001.

Young, Ph.D., Robert O. and Shelly Redford Young. *The pH Miracle: Balance Your Diet, Reclaim Your Health.* Warner Books, Inc., New York: 2002.

INDEX

ABOUT THE AUTHOR

Michelle Schoffro Cook, DNM, DAc, CNC, CITP, is a Doctor of Natural Medicine, Doctor of Acupuncture, Biofeedback Therapist, Holistic Nutritionist, Reiki Master, Energy Medicine Practitioner, and award-winning author. Her studies have taken her around the world to learn some of the best healing techniques of many ancient cultures as well as modern holistic medicine. She received her Doctorate in Acupuncture from the Open International University for Complementary Medicines in Sri Lanka. Having completed over 4,000 hours of training in physical medicine, nutritional and herbal medicine, Eastern natural medicine systems, and homeopathy, she was awarded her Doctor of Natural Medicine designation from the Examining Board of Natural Medicine Practitioners.

Founder and Director of Healing Body, Mind & Spirit in Cochrane, Alberta, Michelle Schoffro Cook has been involved in the healing arts for over fifteen years. Her monthly and bi-monthly columns regularly appear in *Health 'N Vitality*, *Beyond Fitness*, and *Synchronicity* magazines. Schoffro Cook's writing has been featured in over fifty publications worldwide. She is currently completing her third book, *The Ultimate Body Detox Plan* (Wiley, 2005), which is based on many years of research to develop her revolutionary plan to help people overcome disease and experience vibrant health.

Michelle Schoffro Cook has received numerous awards for her writing, including a Crystal Award of Excellence. She was also awarded the prestigious Forty Under 40 Award as one of the top business people and leaders in Canada's Capital Region. She has delivered workshops to both corporate and government audiences from as far away as Beijing, China.

ISBN 141203005-6